The Bicycle Fitness Book

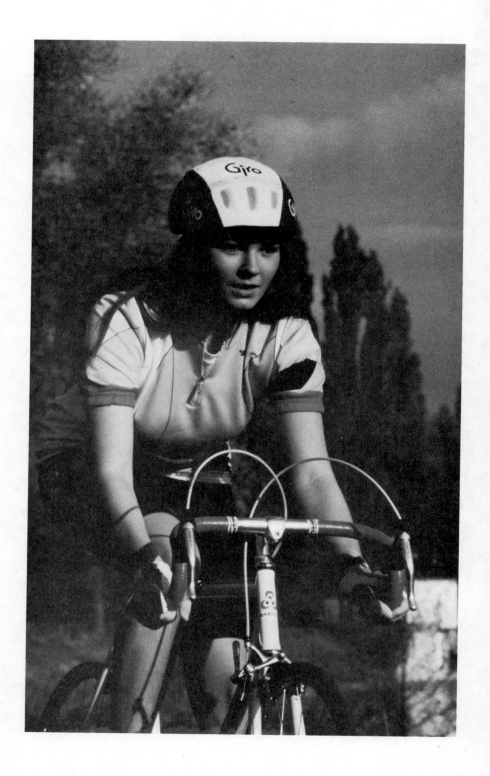

The Bicycle Fitness Book
Riding your bike for health and fitness
Rob Van der Plas

Illustrated by the author

Bicycle Books — San Francisco

Published by :
Bicycle Books, Inc.
P.O.Box 2038
Mill Valley CA 94941
USA

Distributed to the book trade by:
USA: The Talman Company, New York, NY
Canada: Raincoast Book Distribution, Vancouver, BC
UK: Chris Lloyd Sales and Marketing Services, Poole, Dorset

Cover photograph by Neil Van der Plas

Library of Congress Cataloging in Publication Data
Van der Plas, Robert, 1938 —
The Bicycle Fitness Book, Riding your bike for health and fitness, 1989
Includes index
1. Bicycles and Bicycling, Manuals, Handbooks, etc.
2. Authorship, Manuals, Handbooks, etc.
I. Title

Library of Congress Catalog Card Number 89-61366

ISBN 0-933201-23-0 Paperback

Table of Contents

About the Author 6

Part I – Bicycle Basics 7
1. Why Cycle for Fitness? 7
2. Bike Set-up and Basic Riding 11
3. Bike Handling Techniques 18
4. Using the Gears 28
5. Bicycle Safety 34
6. Bicycling Health 39

Part II – Training For Fitness **43**
7. What Makes the Bicycle Go? 43
8. What Makes the Cyclist Go? 48
9. Your Muscles at Work 54
10. Food for Cycling and Fitness 61
11. Improving Your Endurance 69
12. Basic Training Theory 73
13. On-the-Bike Training Methods 83
14. Indoor Training Methods 88
15. Your Personal Training Plan 96

Part III – Know Your Equipment **102**
16. Selecting a Bicycle 102
17. Frame, Steering and Saddle 107
18. The Bicycle's Other Components 114
19. Other Equipment 124
20. Bicycle Clothing 132

Appendix **138**
Table 1 – Frame sizing 138
Table 2 – Gear table 139
Table 3 – Gearing conversion table 139

Index 140

About the Author

Rob Van der Plas is a lifelong bicycle enthusiast and an acknowledged expert in the field. He is the author of numerous books on the subject, including *The Bicycle Racing Guide*, which forms the basis of much of the physiological material included in the present work.

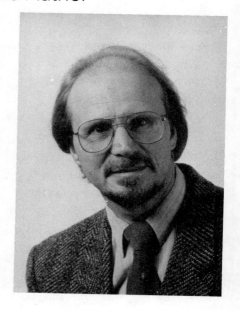

In addition to his numerous books, articles about various aspects of the sport and the technical details of the bicycle written by him regularly appear in specialized periodicals on both sides of the Atlantic.

To Van der Plas, fitness is not necessarily just something to dream of, but something to live. Riding the bicycle regularly for many of his everyday transportation needs, he clocks up 100 miles a week in his regular schedule. This keeps him fit the 'natural way.'

Part I – Bicycle Basics

1. Why Cycle for Fitness?

Bicycle riding is *in*, and so is fitness. But that alone is not necessarily a rational and adequate reason to justify the decision to combine the two. After all, all sorts of things are in fashion at some time or another, but it rarely makes no sense to combine them. Much less to write a book about that mixture. There must be more to cycling for fitness.

Advantages of Cycling

Simply put, there isn't a more suitable method of achieving basic fitness than cycling. And that's not new either. As early as the last quarter of the 19th century, physicians have been commending the bicycle for its unique role in contributing to the people's health — at least where the male population was concerned. Women took a back seat in those days. However healthy cycling may have been for them (and some even doubted that, citing the presumed inherent differences between the two sexes), it was certainly not considered proper for them to do so. In fact, fitness itself seems to have been considered undesirable for women until the dawning of the reform period after the First World War.

Thank goodness those times are over. Today, women outnumber men both amongst runners and cyclists, and a nose count may reveal many other sporting events where women make a strong showing. Fortunately, it does not look as if that will ever turn into the opposite, where some day fitness and physical activity will be considered women's stuff, while men are out taking care of more serious things, getting fat and sluggish in the process.

But back to why the bicycle should be considered the ultimate vehicle in the quest for fitness. In the first place, the bicycle is a useful vehicle — it can be used to get somewhere. So your exercise time is not exclusive: while getting fit, you can get places, see things, and move about at an acceptable rate. Half an hour's cycling can convey a trained cyclist over a distance of 10 miles or more. That way, you can start at the front door and vary the site of the exercise from day to day. And you can do some useful or entertaining things on the way.

A second advantage of cycling is that the body is partially supported, eliminating most of the static loads on the body. And even when you stop pedaling, you neither stop nor fall over. That is the main reason cycling can be maintained for a prolonged period at the desired output level and speed. Whereas half an hour's jogging may seem to take a heavy toll, it is no problem to cycle several hours on end at the same output level.

In the third place, when done correctly — and this book will help you to do so —, cycling does not produce unacceptable loads on joints, muscles, and tendons. This makes cycling possible even when other forms of exercise may be too hard. And it allows cycling to be continued up to a venerable age.

Finally, and to me most importantly, cycling is fun. I think anyone who has learned to cycle effectively will enjoy the speed and silence of propulsion, the graduality and grace of movement, the oneness with the environment that can be enjoyed more in cycling than in any other form of exercise. All in all, there are plenty of good reasons to ride your bike for fitness.

Start Right Here

Though there are another 19 chapters to follow that tell the complete story, there is no need to wait until you've read them all before you start cycling for fitness. Start right here! In this section, I shall describe the very simplest basics of fitness cycling, so you can start getting the benefits and practice what you learn as you read on.

The rest of the book will help you hone your skills and perfect your style. It will help you optimize your training schedule and it will help you understand why you should be doing what. But meanwhile, don't waste all your time reading a book: ride your bike — and do it right, so your quest for fitness and cycling pleasure can start right away.

In a nutshell, the secret of biking for basic fitness is associated with the aerobic training effect. And the secret of aerobic training is that through regular exercise at an output level that is high enough to raise the pulse to a certain level over an adequate period of time, the heart will become stronger and can pump more blood through the veins per heartbeat. This tends to lower the resting pulse — making the heart last longer and its owner live longer.

No ironclad guarantee: if you go about it the wrong way (and reading this book will make sure you don't), you may not benefit. What's worse, done to excess and without proper preparation, too vigorous an exercise may be dangerous. There are plenty of horror stories about sedentary types who try to make up twenty or more years of physical starvation in too short a time, only to suffer a heart attack.

So your first step should be to get a physical examination, pointing out to the physician that you intend to start an aerobic exercise program using the bike. You'll be scrutinized with that in mind and if there are any reservations, you will be told what they are. Thus, you may be told to avoid anaerobic work (sprints, vigorous climbing, etc.). That probably applies to only very few people, but the consequence of ignoring this kind of advice is too great to treat it lightheartedly if it should apply to you.

Once you have a clean bill of health, get something similar for your bike. Take it to the bike shop and have it inspected. Make sure it is adjusted right and in good condition. Then start using it: put it in a low to medium gear and start riding. During the first week, if you have not done much cycling for a long time, it will be smartest to do no more than a couple of miles a day, pedaling at a comfortable rate, just to get used to riding again. After a week or so, start raising the speed and increasing the distance. But for starters, fifteen to twenty minutes of continuous cycling on a regular schedule will do the trick.

Ideally, you should do a trip like this every day of the week. If you have no time or opportunity during the week, the minimum should be Saturday, Sunday and one day midweek, providing you increase the distance (or duration) of the rides by 50%. Wednesday is the best choice for your mid-week ride, since that spaces the effort most effectively — the same advice applies to all more advanced exercises discussed later as well). Try to get to feel at ease on the bike. Practice changing gear, steering, braking, and — even more importantly — looking over your shoulders to see the road is clear before turning off or stopping. Don't push the pedals impulsively but try to spin the legs freely, shifting into a lower gear when you notice too much effort is required to do that in the gear you are in, to a higher one when the resistance is obviously too light.

Once you are at ease on the bike again, or if you are anyway, it will be time to start the simplest schedule of aerobic cycling exercise. Again try to practice as many times a week as you can, but at least three times. Each session will consist of a warming up period, an exertion period and a cooling down period. All you need by way of equipment is a bike and a watch with easy-to-read second hand to monitor your pulse (alternatively, you may use a pulse or heart rate monitoring device, either separate or integrated in a bicycle computer, if you are into fancy gadgetry at all). Manually, you can either check your pulse at the inside of your wrist with the other hand, or you can do it by feeling the carotid artery by the side of the neck, as shown in Fig. 1.1. Count out 15 seconds and multiply by four to get your pulse in beats per minute (bpm).

Your pulse, or heart rate, is the principal guide for determining the intensity of training in any aerobic training program. To calculate the required training pulse, use the following simple formula:

training pulse (bpm) =
180 — your age in years

Keep up this rate for a minimum of 10 minutes if training six times a week, or 20 minutes if you train only three times a week, and you'll be strengthening your heart, improving your condition and making you feel fitter.

But don't forget the other two essential components of your fitness ride: first warm up by cycling at an easy pace for about 5 minutes before you start exert-

ing yourself, and relax the pace for another five minutes afterwards.

Though it may seem blasphemous to some purist in fitness crazes, you needn't go out especially to train: you can do the same thing — either regularly or whenever it suits your schedule — on the way to work, the store or the post office. Use your bike as a means of transportation and it will be much easier to fit cycling for fitness in than when you spend your time twice: the total time needed for a car commute and a separate fitness ride together take a much bigger chunk out of your available time than riding the bike there and back.

And though I will describe the wonderful clothing available to make cycling more comfortable in Chapter 20, it is possible to ride your bike in civies. I'm not telling you to ride around the way cyclists dress in Peking or Amsterdam, nor am I suggesting you use the kind of bike customary there, much less to limit your speed to the 10 mph that is the norm there, but I hope you don't rule out the many other opportunities to use your bike, seeing fitness as a fringe benefit, rather than as your only justification for riding a bicycle.

Cycling with Others

One excellent way to cycle is in the company of others. That can be done informally with friends. But if you take your quest for fitness seriously, it will be necessary to either seek out others with similar goals and conditions, or be prepared to ride alone at least part of the way.

Another fine opportunity is in the form of rides organized by the many cycling clubs around the country. In most urban areas there are several clubs that organize rides for large numbers of participants with a pre-mapped route, but the freedom to establish your own pace. Many of these events are known as Centuries, i.e. 100 mile rides. Or they may be referred to as a metric century,

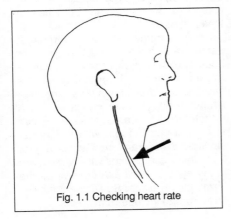

Fig. 1.1 Checking heart rate

i.e. 100km (62 miles). And there are longer rides, too: double and triple centuries are nothing unusual. Watch announcement in the area press for such events or find out directly from the bike clubs.

Although most of these rides are open to all comers, it may well be worthwhile to join a bicycle club. It will certainly improve your cycling skills faster than plodding along alone. It may also be more socially interesting.

A word of warning to the beginner, though. If you have not done any long distance cycling for a long time, don't try to keep up with the gonzos from the bike club. Especially the long distance outings can be very demanding, and it will be much smarter to select your own pace than to try and force a pace that is too high for you. Cycling for basic fitness requires only relatively modest distances, whereas these long rides take more preparation than a couple of 20 minute or even half hour rides. In Part II of the book you will find information about preparing yourself for such events.

About this Book

Allow me to say a few words about the way this book is organized. It consists of three distinct parts and an Appendix. In the first part, you will be familiarized with basic bike set-up and handling, as well as any other essential background information that will help you become a competent cyclist. This includes subjects that range from gearing and braking to health and safety.

In the second part, I shall cover all that is necessary or useful to help you train consciously and effectively. Chapters devoted to the science of cycling and the physiology of the cyclist, to nutrition and to indoor as well as outdoor training methods are included here.

The third part deals with the equipment. There you will learn as much about your bike, the clothes to wear and the other equipment you may want to use as is fit to print.

The Appendix, finally, contains useful reference information that is too prosaic even for the prose form and can be adequately handled only in the form of tables. Here you will find information on frame sizing and gearing.

Choice of Words

This book is distributed both in the US and in other English-speaking countries. Unfortunately, the English language has taken a beating as it traveled across the Atlantic (as the word traveled indicates, which has lost an l on the way over). The difference is not limited to spelling alone. Some words are meaningful only on one side of the big puddle, others have different meanings on either side. Whereas American cyclists ride on somthing they call the pavement, just like American motorists, the English use that word to refer to the part of the road reserved for pedestrians and prams, which in turn are called baby carriages in the US.

Circumstance dictates that I adhere to American spelling wherever the local usage does not stretch the limits of my own tolerance (therefore I shall never plow fields, nor eat donuts or or lite up, using the terms plough, doughnut and light instead). Wherever an American term deviates drastically from its British equivalent, I shall try to explain the word in terms understandable to both the first time it is used.

Finally, another matter of language: gender. As I have as much respect for equality of the sexes as any male can be expected to have, I make a conscious effort to avoid discriminatory language wherever appropriate. However, I have no tolerance for some of the excesses this trend has brought with it. Expressions like *he/she* and *man/woman*, or for that matter compounds with *person*, are in my eyes at least as offensive as the terms they replace. So I'll use the masculin form to include both sexes.

2. Bike Set-up and Basic Riding

This and the following chapters of Part I are primarily devoted to the skills and knowledge that are prerequisite to the safe and enjoyable practice of bicycling, especially as it applies to cycling for fitness. Some of this material may also be found in general bicycle books. However, only here is the practical background of cycling for speed specifically considered.

This particular chapter will first help you arrive at the adjustments that are necessary to cycle in comfort. This is followed by practical advice on posture, riding style and the methods that allow you to cycle continuously at speed. Excluded from this material will be the subject of gearing choice and pedaling rate, since these topics will be covered comprehensively in Chapter 4.

Riding Posture

To cycle fast with endurance, the conventional idea of a comfortable position must be reconsidered. Although bicycle racers have long known that they are most comfortable in a relatively low crouched position, most other cyclists — whatever kind of bike they ride — seem to feel that to be comfortable one has to sit upright. That may be fine for folks who

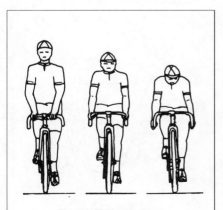

Fig. 2.1 Riding postures

travel only short distances in town or make minor excursions at low speed in easy terrain. However, the serious bicyclist out to improve his fitness level has much more in common with the racer than he has with these occasional short distance cyclists.

Fig. 2.1 shows the three basic kinds of riding posture for comparison: upright, inclined and fully crouched. The cyclist who rides in the upright position may well be convinced this is the only comfortable way to ride a bike. As I look out of my window I see at least thirty people cycling by in this posture each hour. Those who are going north have a very slight uphill — only a 1% slope. All are working hard, you can tell by the strained expression on their faces, their cramped movements and their abysmally slow progress. Every now and again another type of cyclist comes by. Passing the others at twice their speed and obviously more relaxed, these are the ones who ride in either a deep incline or in a fully crouched position.

There are of course also other reasons why the latter are going faster and suffering less, but the first and most important step towards this more comfortable style is their different riding posture. In the lower position, the rider's weight is divided more evenly over handlebars, saddle and pedals. Firstly, this reduces the pressure on the rider's buttocks. Secondly, it allows the relaxed fast pedaling technique so essential for long duration power output. Thirdly, it enables greater restraining forces to bring more force to bear on the pedals.

Finally, it can reduce the wind resistance, which is a major factor in cycling, especially when travelling fast or against the wind regardless of riding speed. The cyclist's frontal area is crucial to the wind resistance, and is much lower in the more inclined positions, which is reflected in the power required to ride the bike at the same speed.

Strangely enough, many people to whom the advantages have been demonstrated nevertheless insist on riding in the upright position. They bring all sorts of arguments, ranging from, "That's only for racing" to, "That is terribly uncomfortable" or, "You couldn't cycle any distance that way." The undeniable fact is that they are fooling themselves. In reality, they are less comfortable, whatever they think, and have to do more work to proceed the same distance or to ride at the same speed. Get accustomed to the right posture early in your cycling career, and you'll be a more effective cyclist, one who gets less frustration and more pleasure out of the pursuit.

If you should think that more effort to have the same effect is a good way to train yourself, you are not only a masochist, you are also fooling yourself. Training in an uncomfortable posture does not tire you out by the physical output, but by the discomfort. In other words, neither your muscles nor your heart or lungs are getting any stronger, though you are suffering without making much progress.

The Basic Posture

Even within the general range of comfortable positions, there are enough different variants to allow changes and adaptations. This makes it possible to adapt to different conditions and gives you the chance to vary your position from time to time. The latter helps avoid the numbing feeling when pressure is applied in the same position for a longer period. Especially the position of the hands may require some variation, certainly if the cyclist is not yet used to supporting a significant portion of his own weight on the arms.

The following sections will describe just how the saddle and the handlebars should be set to achieve the basic relaxed position that is shown in Fig. 2.2. This particular posture is worth looking into a little closer. Study the proportions, noting also that merely holding the handlebars in a different location allows adequate variation. This may be required to apply more force to the pedals or to reduce the wind resistance by lowering the front, or to get a better overview of the road or the scenery by raising the front by as little as perhaps 10cm (4 in) either way. The following description is based on the assumption that you

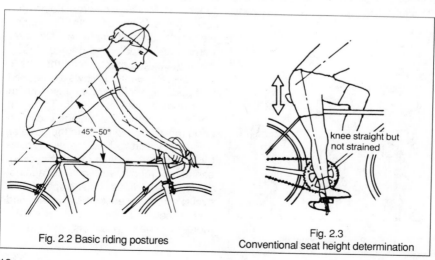

Fig. 2.2 Basic riding postures

Fig. 2.3
Conventional seat height determination

45°–50°

knee straight but not strained

have a drop handlebar derailleur bicycle of the right size to match your physique and a crank length that equals one half the upper leg length.

Saddle Height

The height of the saddle, or rather the distance of its top relative to the pedals, is the most critical variable for effective cycling. It should be adjusted so that the leg can be stretched comfortably without completely stretching the knee, which would force excessive force and rotation on the joint. At the same time, the distance between the pedal in its highest point and the saddle must be such that the knee is not bent excessively. Once the former has been set, the correct crank length, as established in Chapter 18, assures that the latter condition is also satisfied.

Here I shall describe three methods of establishing the correct seat height. These are all good enough for preliminary set-up and the first thousand miles of cycling. Your ultimate seat position may require additional individual experimental fine-tuning, based on your subjective long-term comfort. On the other hand, in the vast majority of all cases, each of these techniques will lead to a satisfactory seat position that is suitable for touring, without the need for subsequent fine-tuning.

The first method is illustrated in Fig. 2.3. You should wear cycling shoes with flat heels. Place the bike next to a wall or post for support when you sit on it. Adjust the seat up or down (following the adjustment procedure below) until it is set at such a height relative to the pedal that the heel of your cycling shoe rests on the pedal when your knee is straight but not strained, with the pedal down, crank in line with the seat tube.

Sit on the bike and place the heels on the pedals. Symmetrical pedals can be merely turned upside down; on platform models the toeclips must be removed. Pedal backwards this way, making sure you do not have to rock from side to side to reach the pedals. Now raise the saddle 12mm (^{1}/2 in) above this height. Tighten the saddle in this position. Note that the heels-on- pedals style only applies to adjusting the seat height, not to riding the bike, as described below.

The second method is referred to as 109% rule. It was developed at Loughborough University in England and is illustrated in Fig. 2.4 To use this method, first measure your inseam leg length by standing with your back against a wall with the legs straight, the feet about 5cm (2 in) apart, wearing thin soled shoes with flat heels. Make a pencil mark for the location of the crotch on the wall. This is easiest to do with the aid of a drawing triangle (oddly enough called a square in Britain) or a rectangular board held upright and pushed up against the wall between the legs. Measure the vertical distance between this mark and the floor.

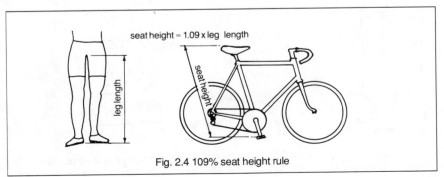

seat height = 1.09 x leg length

Fig. 2.4 109% seat height rule

Now multiply the figure so found by 1.09. That is presumed to be the optimal distance between the top of the saddle and the pedal axle when the pedal is down, crank in line with the seat tube. Measure it out and set the seat accordingly with the plane connecting front and back of the saddle cover horizontal. How the saddle is raised or lowered will be explained below.

The third method, illustrated in Fig. 2.5, was developed by the American bicycle racing coach Mark Hodges. It is probably the most accurate method, applicable to fitness cyclists as much as it is to racers. You will need a helper to measure your leg length and a calculator to figure out the correct saddle height. Stand barefoot upright with your back against a wall, the feet 15 cm (6 in) apart. Now measure the distance from the floor over the ankle joint and the knee joint to the greater trochanter. That's the outwardmost bump on the femur or hip, which coincides with the hip joint's center of rotation: when you raise the leg this point does not move.

To establish the optimal seat height, measured between the top of the saddle near its center and the center of the pedal axle (crank pointing down in line with the seat tube), multiply the dimension so found by 0.96. If appropriate, add an allowance for thick soles, thick cleats or special clipless pedals with matching shoes.

Even after using any of these methods, you may have to do some fine-tuning to achieve long-term comfort. Riders with disproportionately small feet may want to place the saddle a little lower, those with big feet perhaps slightly higher. No need to get carried away: raise or lower the seat in steps of 6mm ($^1/4$ in) at a time and try to get used to any position by riding several hundred miles or at least a week before attempting any change, which must again be in the order of about 6 mm to make any real difference.

When cycling, the ball of the foot (the second joint of the big toe) should be over the center of the pedal axle, with the heel raised so much that the knee is never straightened fully. Not all cyclists incline the foot equally; consequently, the amount by which the saddle is moved relative to the point determined may vary a little for different riders — a matter of 6mm ($^1/4$ in) one way or the other.

Saddle Position and Angle

The normal preliminary saddle position is such that the seat post is roughly in the middle of the saddle. For optimal

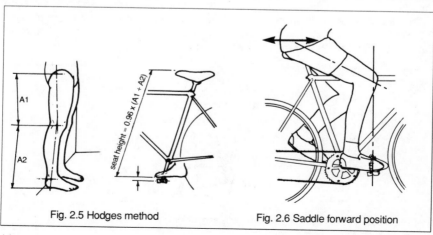

Fig. 2.5 Hodges method

Fig. 2.6 Saddle forward position

pedaling efficiency, adjust the saddle forward or backwards after it has been set to the correct height, as explained in the preceding section. On any bike designed on conventional lines, sitting on the bike with the foot under the toeclip and the crank placed horizontally, the center of the knee joint must be vertically aligned with the spindle of the forward pedal, as shown in Fig. 2.6.

The angle of the saddle relative to the horizontal plane should initially be set so as to keep the line that connects the highest points at the front and the back level. After the handlebars have been set to the correct height, it may be necessary to modify this angle to prevent slipping forward or backwards. This too may not become apparent until after some miles of cycling. Adjusting procedures for both forward position and angle are outlined below.

Saddle Adjustments

To do the actual mechanical adjusting work on the saddle, first take a close look at the way it is installed on the bike, comparing it with Fig. 17.11 in Part III of the book. The saddle height is adjusted by loosening the binder bolt behind the seat lug, raising or lowering the saddle with the attached seat post in a twisting motion, and then tightening the binder bolt again at the required height, making sure it is straight.

To change the forward position, undo the adjustment bolts (only one bolt on some models) on your adjustable seat post. These bolts are usually reached from under the saddle cover, though they can be reached from below or the side on some models. Once loosened, push the saddle forward or backwards until the desired position is reached; then tighten the bolts, making sure the saddle is held under the desired angle relative to the horizontal plane.

Handlebar Height and Position

The highest point of the handlebars should always be lower than the top of the saddle to ride efficiently. Just how low will be determined by the shape of the handlebars and the rider's physiognomy. It depends on the relative distribution of body weight and torso height, as well as on the upper and lower arm length. That's why only experiments can tell what will eventually be right for any particular rider. Here I shall merely tell you how to determine the initial position for a relaxed initial riding style. After about a thousand miles of cycling, you should be able to fine- tune the handlebar height and stem length to match your needs perfectly.

The following description is again based on the use of a correctly dimensioned frame, as outlined in Chapter 17. In order to make sure it is not too high, first check whether the fully crouched position can be achieved. Place the handlebars in their lowest possible position and, sitting on the saddle, hold them in the lowest part of the bend (below the brake levers). With the lower arms horizontal and the elbows under a slightly acute angle, the upper body should now lie almost horizontally. This is the fully crouched or 'full tuck' position. It may be necessary to choose a longer or shorter handlebar stem for comfort in this position. If this full tuck is not possible with any handlebar stem available, a smaller or (more rarely) a larger frame may be required.

To set the handlebars for a relaxed initial riding style, without sacrificing the advantages of the full tuck when conditions call for it, proceed as follows. First set the top of the bars about 3cm ($1\frac{1}{4}$ in) lower than the saddle. Sit on the bike and reach forward for the part of the bends between the straight top and the brake handle attachments. In this position your shoulders should be about midway between seat and hands, as shown in Fig. 2.2. The arms should feel neither stretched nor heavily loaded and they should run parallel.

If they don't satisfy the last criterion, your handlebar bend is too wide or too narrow; if you can not find a relaxed position, you will need a longer or shorter stem. If you should have a particularly long combination of lower arms and torso in relation to your leg length, you may not be comfortable even with a long stem. In that case, a slightly larger frame, which has a longer top tube as well as a longer seat tube, may be in order. Conversely, long legs combined with short arms and torso may require you use a shorter frame to achieve the right top tube length. In extreme cases of either variety, the right top tube length just cannot be achieved with a bike that fits in height. In this case, you may need a custom-built frame with the desired dimensions of seat tube and top tube. This would be the ultimate solution, although it is probably not quite so critical that you can't make do with a stock frame.

Finally, grab the handlebar bend at the ends, leaning forward on them while seated. The handlebar angle relative to the horizontal plane should be such that the hands don't slip either into the bend or off towards the ends in this position. If you initially have difficulties achieving this position, you may start off with the handlebars somewhat higher. In that case, the ends must also point down slightly. Lower and level them out as you develop the style that allows you to ride with the lower handlebar position after some practice.

Handlebar Adjustments

To vary the height of the handlebars, straddle the front wheel, facing the bike. Undo the expander bolt, which is recessed in the top of the stem (refer to Fig.17.9 inPart III). If the stem does not come loose immediately, you may have to lift the handlebars to raise the wheel off the ground, then tap on the head of

the expander bolt with a hammer. This will loosen the internal clamping device. Now raise or lower the handlebar stem as required. Tighten the expander bolt again, while holding the handlebars straight in the desired position.

To change the angle of the handlebar ends with respect to the horizontal plane, undo the binder bolt that clamps the handlebar bend in the front of the stem. Twist the handlebar bend until it is under the desired angle, and then tighten the binder bolt again, holding the bar centered. To install a longer stem or a different bar design, you are referred to any bicycle maintenance book or your friendly bike store. The correct handlebar position often puts more strain on the hands than beginning cyclists find comfortable, especially when rough road surfaces induce vibrations. Minimize this problem by always keeping the arms slightly bent, never holding them in a cramped position. If you still experience discomfort, wrap the handlebars with cushioned foam sleeves (such as Grab-On) instead of normal handlebar tape.

Adjusting Mountain Bikes

For those who use a mountain bike or a hybrid bike, most of the adjustments described above also apply as long as you ride on the road. Since most of your riding will probably be done on the road, whatever kind of bike is used, the only real difference is that the flat mountain bike handlebars do not allow the lower position for the full tuck. Consequently, I suggest you set the saddle and the handlebars so that the relaxed position described above is possible when holding the flat bars at the ends.

Basic Bike Handling

Once saddle and handlebars are adjusted correctly, it will be time to take to the road on your bike. In case you are not yet familiar with the derailleur bicycle and the rest of your equipment, here's just a suggestion for getting on and off the bike. All other riding and handling techniques involve long learning processes that will be treated in separate chapters, but the simple act of starting the bike should be mastered immediately.

Before you start off, make sure your shoe laces are tied and tucked in, or short enough not to run the risk of getting caught in the chain. Put the bike in a low gear.

Start off at the side of the road, after having checked to make sure no traffic is following closely behind. Straddle the top tube by swinging the appropriate leg either over the handlebars, the top tube, or the saddle. Hold the handlebars with both hands at the top of the bend. Tap against the pedal with the toe of your starting foot to turn it around. This brings the toeclip or the clipless binding on top, after which you can immediately insert the foot. Pedal backward until the pedal is in the top position if you use toeclips, then pull the toe strap, but not quite so tight as to cut off circulation in the foot, then pedal back three quarters of a revolution to bring the pedal to 2 o'clock, just above the horizontally forward position. Don't tuck in the ends of the toestraps. If you have clipless pedals with matching shoes, learn and practice how the particular model used is inserted and removed.

Look behind you to make sure the road is clear, then check ahead to establish which course you'll want to follow. Place your weight on the pedal, leaning lightly on the handlebars. Put the other foot on its pedal as soon as it is in the top position. When you have gained some momentum, tap the toe against the back of the free pedal to turn it over, and right away slide the foot in under the toeclip. Pedal a few more strokes, then pull the loose toestrap taut, securing the second foot to its pedal as well.

To slow down, whether just to stop or to get off the bike, first look behind you again to make sure you are not getting in the way of cyclists or motorists following. Aim for the position where you will want to stop. Change into a lower gear, appropriate for starting off again later. Push against the buckle of the toestrap for whichever foot you want to have free first (or liberate your foot from the clipless patent pedal, if that is what you use), meanwhile pulling the foot up and back to loosen it when that pedal is up.

Slow down by braking gently, using mainly the front brake to stop. When you have come to a standstill, or just before that point, make sure the pedal with the loosened strap is up, then pull the foot up and out. Place it on the ground, leaning over in the same direction, while moving forward off the saddle to straddle the top tube. Now you are in the right position to dismount or start again.

If you want to get off the bike at this point, bring the other foot up, pedaling backwards, and loosen the clipless binding or the toestrap to release the foot. Now you're ready to get off the bike. However, under most circumstances you will find that the machine is most easily controlled when you remain on the bike, straddling the top tube. Consequently, I suggest you only dismount completely if it is really necessary.

3. Bike Handling Techniques

In the present chapter, we will take a closer look at the skills needed to ride the bicycle effectively and safely. Though other cyclists — be they tourers or commuters — also have to master similar skills, there are some special aspects to consider for cycling at speed, which will be emphasized here wherever appropriate.

The first section of this chapter will deal with honing your skills of riding the bicycle competently, with proper control over the steering and braking mechanisms. This will help you cycle with minimal effort and maximum confidence. In the next section you will be introduced to the peculiarities of effective riding techniques for cycling at speed. Although an understanding of the theoretical background is helpful, I shall concentrate as much as possible on the practical aspects, making you practice what you learn.

The Steering Principle
A bicycle is not steered most effectively by merely turning the handlebars and following the front wheel, as is the case for any two-track vehicle, such as a car. Though bicycles and other single-track vehicles indeed follow the front wheel, they also require the rider to lean his

vehicle into the curve to balance it at the same time.

If you were to merely turn the handlebars, the lower part of the bike would start running away from its previous course in the direction in which the front wheel is then pointed. Meanwhile, the mass of the rider, perched high up on the bike, would continue following the original course due to inertia. Thus, the center of gravity would not be in line with the supporting bike, and the rider would come crashing to the ground. Due to the effect of centrifugal force, the tendency to throw the rider off towards the outside of the curve increases with higher speeds, requiring a more pronounced lean the faster you are going.

It is possible to steer by turning the handlebars, and then correct lean and steering to regain balance afterwards. In fact, many older people, especially women, seem to do it that way, succeeding quite well at low speeds only. As soon as imbalance becomes imminent, they have to make a correction in the other direction. After some cramped and anxious movements, they finally get around the corner. This accounts for the tensioned and apparently impulsive riding style typical for such riders, even if they have practiced it so long that they

Curve radius, speed and lean are inter-related. At higher speed, more lean in the direction of the turn is required. The figure in the center follows the natural curve. To force a tighter curve at a low speed, lean the bike more than the body. To force a tighter curve at high speed, lean the body more than the bike.

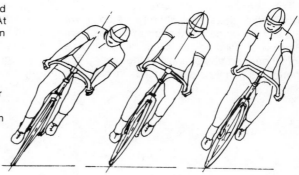

Fig. 3.1 Bike and body lean in curve

don't realize their movements are awkward and their balance precarious.

The more effective technique for riding a curve at speed is based on placing the bike under the appropriate angle, where the centrifugal force is offset by a shift of the mass center to the inside, before turning off. Two methods may be used, depending on the amount of time and room available to carry out the maneuver. I refer to these two methods as natural and forced turn, respectively. To understand either, we should first take a look at the intricacies of balancing the bike when riding a straight line, after which the two methods of turning can be explained.

Bicycle Balance

What keeps a bicycle or any other single track vehicle going without falling over is the inertia of its moving mass. Rolling a narrow hoop will show that it is an unstable balance: once the thing starts to lean either left or right, it will just go down further and further until it hits the ground. That's because the mass is no longer supported vertically in line with the force. Try it with a bicycle wheel if you like. If the bike's front wheel could not be steered and the rider couldn't move sideways, he'd come down the same way very soon.

On the bicycle, the rider feels when the vehicle starts to lean over. Theoretically, there are two ways out of the predicament: either move the rider back over the center of the bike or move the bike back under the rider. In practice, the latter method is used most effectively, especially at higher speeds. When the bike begins leaning to the side, the rider oversteers the front wheel a little in the same direction, which places the bike back in such a position that balance is restored. In fact, this point will be passed, so the bike starts leaning over the other way, and so on.

This entire sequence of movements is relatively easy to notice when you are cycling slowly. When standing still, the balancing motions are so extreme that only a highly skilled cyclist can keep control. The faster the bicycle, the less perceptible (though equally important and therefore harder to master) are the steering corrections required to retain balance. To get an understanding of this whole process, I suggest you practice riding a straight line at a low speed. Then do it at a higher speed, and see whether you agree with the explanation, referring also to Fig. 3.1.

Both riding a straight line and staying upright with the bike are merely illusions. In reality, the bike is always in disequilibrium, following a more or less curved track. The combination of bike with rider leans alternately one way and the other. At higher speeds the curves are longer and gentler, while the amount of lean can be perceptible; at lower speeds the curves are shorter and sharper, with less pronounced lean angles for any given deviation.

The Natural Turn

Under normal circumstances, the rider knows well ahead where to turn off, and there is enough room to follow a generously wide curve. This is the situation of the natural turn. It makes use of the lean that results from normal straight path steering corrections. To turn to the right naturally, you simply wait until the bike is leaning over that way, while the left turn is initiated when the bike is leaning to the left.

Instead of turning the handlebars to that same side, as would be done to get back in balance to ride straight, you just leave the handlebars alone for a while. This causes the bike to lean over further and further in the direction of the turn. Only when the lean is quite significant, do you steer in the same direction, but not as abruptly as you would do to get back up straight. Instead, you fine-tune the ratio of lean and steering deflection to ride the curve out.

When the turn is completed, you will still be leaning over in the direction of the turn, and you would ride a circle without some other corrective action on your part. You get back on the straight course by steering further into the curve than the amount of lean demands to maintain your balance. This puts your mass center back right above the bike or even further over, allowing you to resume the slightly curving course with which you approximate the straight line. This is illustrated in Fig. 3.2.

Chances are you learned to do this subconsciously when you were a kid, but never realized that you were doing all this. You could perhaps continue to ride a bicycle forever without understanding the theory. However, to keep control over the bike in demanding situations encountered while riding fast in difficult terrain, you will be much better off if you have the theoretical knowledge and have learned to ride a calculated course, making use of this information. Get a feel for it by riding around an empty parking lot many times, leaning this way and that, following straight lines and making turns, until it is both second nature and something you can do consciously, knowing the relevant limitations.

While you are practicing this techni-que, as well as when riding at other times, note that speed, curve radius, lean and load are all closely correlated. A sharper turn requires more lean at any given speed. At a higher speed, any given curve requires much greater lean angles than the same curve radius at a lower speed. Finally, the loaded bike tends to lean more than an unloaded machine. As you practice this technique, learn to judge which are the appropriate combinations under different circumstances.

The Forced Turn

You will often be confronted with situations that don't allow you to wait until you are conveniently leaning the appropriate way to make a gradual turn. Deficiencies in the road surface or the presence of other traffic in the road may force you into a narrow predetermined path, with only a few inches to deviate sideways. Or a sudden obstacle may force you to divert suddenly. Finally, you may have to get around a curve that is too sharp to be taken naturally at your current riding speed.

These situations require the second method of turning, illustrated in Fig. 3.3, which I call the forced turn. In this case, the turn must be initiated quickly, regardless which way the bike happens to be

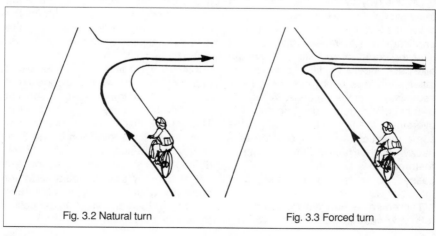

Fig. 3.2 Natural turn   Fig. 3.3 Forced turn

leaning at the time. You have to force the bike to lean over in the appropriate direction and under the right angle consistent with the direction and radius of the turn. And it has to be done quickly.

Do that by sharply steering away from the turn just before you get there. You and the bike will immediately start to lean over in the direction of the turn. You would risk a disastrous crash, as your bike moves away precipitously from the mass center, if you were to continue in a straight line. You have very quickly achieved a considerable lean angle in the direction of the turn. This must be compensated by steering quite abruptly in the same direction. Since this is the direction of the turn, you are set up just right to make a sharp turn. Once completed, steer back into the turn just a little further, to get the lean for regaining the roughly straight course, as explained for the natural turn.

The forced turn technique should be practiced intensely and consciously, since it by no means comes naturally. Initiating a left turn by steering right will probably require the beginning cyclists to overcome all sorts of reasonable inhibitions and demands lots of practice. Take your bike to a grassy area or an empty parking lot a few days in a row, wearing protective clothing in case you fall: helmet, gloves, jacket and long pants.

Practice and experiment until you've mastered the trick, and refresh your skill from time to time, until this instant turning technique has become second nature. The forced turn will not only be helpful when taking a tight turn, but is of equal benefit when you need to temporarily divert from your straight course for one reason or the other. In a subsequent section of this chapter you will be shown how to apply it to the difficult task of avoiding a suddenly appearing obstacle.

Braking Technique

Any cyclist sometimes has to use the brakes, though not always to make a panic stop. In fact, the sensible cyclist should hardly ever have to brake to a standstill. Instead, you will be using the brakes to control and regulate your speed.

Effective braking means that you can ride up fast close to the turn or the obstacle which requires the reduced speed, brake to reach the lower speed quickly, and accelerate immediately afterwards. So you will be using the brakes to get down in speed from 30 to 20 MPH to take a turn, or from 30 to 28 MPH to avoid running into the person ahead of you. Or you may have to get down from 50 to 10 MPH to handle a switchback or hairpin curve on a steep descent. To do that effectively without risk requires an understanding of braking physics. Though at times you may have to reduce speed quickly, you should also develop a feel for gradual speed reduction to prevent skidding and loss of control. In fact, most cyclists are more often in danger due to braking too vigorously than due to insufficient stopping power.

Braking amounts to deceleration or speed reduction, which can only take place gradually. The rate of deceleration can be measured and is expressed in m/sec^2. A deceleration of $1 m/sec^2$ means that after each second of braking the travelling speed is 1 m/sec less than it was at the beginning of that second. A speed of 30 MPH corresponds to 13m/sec. To get down to standstill would take 13 sec, if the braking deceleration is 1m/sec; it would take 4 seconds to reach 9m/sec or 20 MPH. At a higher rate of deceleration it would take less time (and a shorter distance) to get down to the desired speed.

The modern derailleur bicycle has remarkably effective brakes, providing it's not raining. A modest force on the brake handle can cause a deceleration of 4—5m/sec^2 with just one brake. Applying both brakes, the effect is even more dramatic, enabling you to slow down from 30 to 15 MPH within one second. There are some limitations to braking that have to be considered, though.

In the first place, rain has a negative effect on the rim brake's performance, as the build-up of water on the rims reduces the friction between brake block and rim drastically. This applies especially if the thing is equipped with ordinary rubber brake blocks, as offered by most manufacturers as standard equipment. With any rubber brake blocks, I measured a reduction from 4.5 to 2.0m/sec^2 for a given lever force (and to half that figure for bicycles with chrome plated steel rims, which should therefore not be used, even on the cheap bicycles on which they are installed). Lately, some special brake block materials have been introduced that are less sensitive to rain.

The second restriction is associated with a change in the distribution of weight between the wheels as a result of braking. Because the mass center of the rider is quite high above the road, and its horizontal distance to the front wheel axle comparatively small, the bicycle has a tendency to tip forward in response to deceleration. Weight is transferred from the rear to the front of the bike, as illustrated in Fig. 3.4. When the deceleration reaches about 3.5m/sec^2, the weight on the rear wheel is no longer enough to provide traction, and the contact between tire and road is reduced to zero. Braking harder than that with the rear brake just makes the rear wheel skid, resulting in loss of control.

In a typical riding posture, the rear wheel actually starts to lift off the ground when a deceleration of about 6.5m/sec^2 is reached, whether using both brakes together or the front brake alone. Consequently, no conventional bicycle can ever be decelerated beyond this limit, regardless of the kind, number and quality of the brakes. This is a very high deceleration, which you should not often reach, but it is good to realize there is such a limit and that it can not be avoided by using the rear brake either alone or in addition to the front brake, but only by braking less vigorously. During a sudden speed reduction or panic stop such high decelerations may be reached. On a downslope the effect will be even more pronounced, since it raises the rider even higher relative to the front wheel. In all such cases, reduce the toppling-over effect by shifting your body weight back and down as much as possible: sit far back and hold the upper body horizontally.

Since about twice as great a deceleration is possible with the front brake as with the one in the rear, the former should be preferably used under most conditions. In most circumstances short of a panic stop or braking in a curve, you can brake very effectively using the front brake alone. When both brakes are used simultaneously, the one in the front can be applied quite a bit harder than the one in the rear. If you notice the rear brake is less effective if pressed equally far, it will be time to check, and if necessary adjust, lubricate or replace the brake cable.

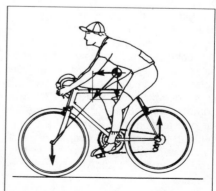

Fig. 3.4 Weight transfer during braking

Of course, most braking is not done abruptly, so gradual braking must also be practiced. In particular when the road is slick, in curves or when others are following closely behind, gradual deceleration and the ability to control the braking force within narrow limits is of vital importance. Practice braking consciously with utmost attention to the complex relationship between initial speed, brake lever force and deceleration, to become fully competent at handling the bike when slowing down under all conceivable circumstances.

Braking becomes a different kettle of fish in hilly terrain. On a steep downhill, the slope not only increases the tendency to tip forward, it also induces an accelerating effect, which must be overcome by the brakes even to merely keep the speed constant. A 20% slope, which is admittedly rarely encountered, induces an acceleration of about $2m/sec^2$. Obviously, you will encounter big problems in wet weather on such a downhill stretch if you don't keep your speed down to start with. So it will be necessary to reduce the speed by gradual, intermittent braking. This will help wipe most of the water from the rims, retaining braking efficiency a little better. This way, the brakes are not overtaxed when you do have to reduce the speed suddenly, as may be required to handle an unexpected obstacle or a sharp turn.

General Riding Techniques

Riding a derailleur bicycle with total confidence requires hands-on experience. That is one good reason to ride lots of miles before you go on longer rides with others. But some of the associated skills can be learned faster and more thoroughly when you understand the principles that are applied. Building up on the information about posture, steering and braking provided in this and the preceding chapter, you will be shown here what to do under various typical riding situations.

Getting up to Speed

Especially for the fitness cyclist, it is important to know how to reach an acceptable speed quickly and smoothly. In Chapter 2, you have been shown how to get on the bike and start off smoothly. The next trick is to reach the ultimate riding speed as quickly and efficiently as possible. The idea is to waste as little time and energy as possible during this process of getting up to speed. Tricky, because acceleration demands disproportionately high levels of power and consumes energy correspondingly. And the faster it's done, the more demanding it is.

Clearly, you have to strike a balance here. Accelerating faster than necessary wastes energy that will be sorely needed later. Done too slowly, it may become a plodding affair. It will be your decision to find the right balance between speed and power, but the way to reach it is easy to describe: start in a low gear and increase speed gradually but rapidly. No fast and slow spurts but a gradual build-up of speed.

Either keep pedaling faster and faster in the low gear, changing up only as you reach a significant speed, or be prepared to do some short duration hard work, standing on the pedals, pulling on the upstroke, as well as pushing on the downstroke. As soon as speed is reached, sit on the saddle and select a good gear for spinning at a comfortable but high pedaling rate.

Riding a Constant Speed

With a small measuring device called accelerometer, one can follow the changes in riding speed of a cyclist travelling at speed. It has been found that the most effective riders tend to be those whose speed varies least over time. Not only does a good cyclist ride the same number of miles one hour as the next, he travels as many yards one minute as the next, as many feet with one crank revolution as the next, and indeed ideally as many inches during each section within any revolution. If you slow down during one short section, it will take disproportionately more time and energy to make up for the loss.

Pay attention to this at all times while cycling. As long as the external conditions don't change drastically, you should make every effort to keep a constant speed and movement. Gauge your speed by comparing it to that of your companions, or use your watch, counting out pedal revolutions and milestones when cycling alone.

Accelerating

However efficient a constant speed may be, sometimes you will still want to accelerate to a higher speed. This may be necessary to add sprinting skills and power to your training schedule or for a more practical reason, such as to catch up with riders ahead, so you can take advantage of the wind-breaking effect by riding immediately behind them, or to avoid getting dropped behind. In traffic, you may have to accelerate in situations like getting across an intersection before the light changes or to avoid running into another vehicle crossing your path.

As with getting up to speed in the first place, it is most efficient to increase the speed as gradually as possible. Unless you are already spinning at your highest possible rate, you will find accelerating by increasing pedaling speed more effective than by increasing pedal force in a higher gear. In other words, as long as you can spin faster, it is best to shift down into a slightly lower gear and increase the pedaling rate vigorously. Once you are gathering momentum and are getting close to your maximum spinning speed, shift up and continue to gain speed in the slightly higher gear.

Riding Against the Wind

At higher speeds or whenever there is a head wind, the effect of air drag on the power needed to cycle is quite significant. Economize on your effort by avoiding the wind resistance as much as possible. Keep your profile as low as possible when cycling against the wind. Especially when riding alone, try to seek out the sheltered parts of the road wherever possible, without exposing yourself to danger.

When you ride in a group, try to exploit the wind shelter effect of riding immediately behind another rider, or staggered appropriately when there is a

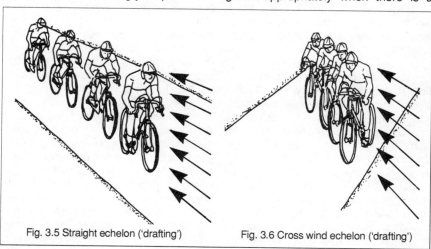

Fig. 3.5 Straight echelon ('drafting')   Fig. 3.6 Cross wind echelon ('drafting')

cross wind. This technique is referred to as drafting in the US or pacing in Britain. Figures 3.5 and 3.6 show the resulting configurations for situations without and with cross wind, respectively.

Hill Climbing

Climbing uphill by bike is not just another skill that can be learned equally well by all, it also requires a certain physique for greatest effectiveness. With some conscious effort, everybody's climbing skills can be improved up to a point; yet some riders are born climbers, while others may have to go uphill slowly all their lives. What it takes is a high power to weight ratio. To put it differently, you need a big heart and voluminous lungs relative to the total body mass. In general, a low body weight will be advantageous. Just the same, it is an ability that can be learned and developed well enough by the average rider to at least handle all hills you encounter, even if you go up slowly.

Again, a regular motion is most efficient, and that is best mastered by staying seated in a rather low gear. For a hilly tour, you should take the trouble to equip the bike with wider ratio gearing than for level riding. Just what sizes of sprockets should be installed is up to you, but I'd say 90% of all beginners tend to pick gear ratios that are too high (or, to put it differently, sprockets that are too small). For mountainous terrain, there should be nothing embarrassing about a rear sprocket with 30 teeth and a chainwheel with 36 or even fewer teeth in the back.

Some bikes, and particularly mountain bikes, are equipped with gears that are low enough to tackle almost any hill without having to get up from the saddle. And on these bikes we sometimes see the other extreme: people riding in gears that are far too low for the circumstances, spinning like mad but getting nowhere fast. Ride in a gear that allows you to spin fast but with noticeable resistance, so your progress is not merely

limited by the speed with which you can turn your legs but by total output.

Climbing out of the Saddle

When the lowest available gear is too high to allow a smoothly spinning leg motion, it is time to shift to another technique. Some riders try to increase the length of the power stroke by means of some hefty ankle twisting, really pushing the leg around at this point. That is an unnecessarily tiring technique, requiring long muscle work phases and short recovery periods. A better method of climbing in a high gear and at a low pedaling speed is referred to as 'honking' in Britain, and seems to be a mystery to most American cyclists.

Honking makes use of the rider's body weight to push down the pedals, while the body is pulled up after each stroke very quickly by standing up. In this mode, the muscle work is done each time the body is raised, rather than when pushing the pedal down and around. To do it effectively, hold the tops of the brake handle mounts in the front of the handlebars. You can either take quick snappy steps or throw your weight from side to side in a swinging motion, as illustrated in Fig. 3.7. I suggest you prac-

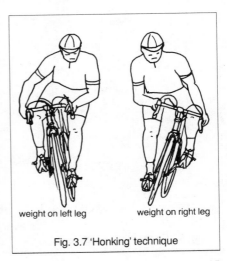

weight on left leg   weight on right leg

Fig. 3.7 'Honking' technique

tice honking as well as spinning: the one in a high gear at pedaling speeds below 55 RPM, the other in a low gear at 65 RPM or more. Avoid pedaling rates of 55—65 RPM by choosing the gearing range to stay within either the one range or the other.

Avoiding Obstacles

Sometimes you will be confronted with some kind of obstacle right in your path. This may be anything from a pothole or a broken branch to a discarded can or bottle. Even when travelling at speed and with little room to maneuver, you can learn to avoid running into such things by using the technique of the forced turn illustrated in Fig. 3.8.

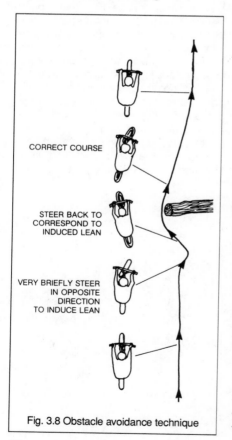

CORRECT COURSE

STEER BACK TO CORRESPOND TO INDUCED LEAN

VERY BRIEFLY STEER IN OPPOSITE DIRECTION TO INDUCE LEAN

Fig. 3.8 Obstacle avoidance technique

As soon as you perceive the obstacle ahead of you, decide whether to pass it to the left or the right. Fix your sight on the point where you intend to pass, rather than on the obstacle itself. Ride straight up to it and then, before you reach it, briefly but decisively steer into the direction opposite to that of your chosen avoidance (to the right if you want to pass on the left). This makes the bike lean over towards the other side (to the left in this case). Now steer in that direction just as quickly, which will result in a very sharp forced turn. As soon as you've passed the obstacle, oversteer a little more, to cause a lean that helps you put the bike back on its proper course.

This too is something to practice on an empty parking lot, wearing a helmet and two long sleeved shirt (the double layer of fabric is much easier on the skin, since the one layer will just slip off the other, rather than removing chunks of your flesh). Mark phoney obstacles with chalk or place foam pads or sponges on the pavement, and practice passing them abruptly on both sides until you've mastered the trick.

Jumping the Bike

Another useful act for hard riding situations is the skill of making first the front, then the rear wheel jump over an obstacle. You may have to do that when there is an unavoidable obstacle ahead of you. It's a matter of shifting your weight back or forth to lift the appropriate wheel off the ground. To jump up, first throw your weight backwards, while pulling up on the handlebars to unload the front wheel while lifting it. At the same time accelerate vigorously, by pushing hard on the forward pedal. With some practice, you'll soon be able to lift the front end of the bike at least a foot up in the air.

Next, try to do the same with the rear wheel, throwing your weight forward while pulling up your legs and bottom at the same time. This is harder, but it can also be mastered. Finally, practice coordinating the two shifts, so that you first lift the front and then, as soon as you've reached the highest point, start raising the back. After some time, you should be able to actually make the bike fly: lift both wheels in such short sequence that the rear wheel comes off the ground well before the front wheel comes down.

One variant of this technique is the art of jumping up sideways, which may be needed to handle obstacles like curbs, ridges and tracks that run nearly parallel to the road. To do this, the bike has to be forced to move sideways in a short and snappy diversion just preceding the jump. Do that by combining the diversion technique described above under *Avoiding Obstacles* with the jump.

Get close to the ridge you want to jump, riding parallel to it. Then briefly steer away from the ridge. This immediately causes the bike to lean towards the obstacle. Now catch yourself by steering sharply in that same direction, lifting the front wheel when you are close to the obstacle, immediately followed by the rear wheel. Practice is all it takes, and the empty parking lot with a chalk line as a substitute ridge is the best place to do that.

Sometimes, you will have to ride through a big pothole, a ditch or any other depression. To do that with minimal risk to bike and rider, you can use something akin to the jumping technique. Enter the depression with your weight near the front of the bike. Then unload the front wheel by throwing your weight back and pulling up the handlebars, just before the front wheel hits the lowest point of the depression. Finally,

ride up the other side and pull up the rear, while shifting your weight to the front of the bike to climb back out. This technique is particularly useful when cycling off-road. In open terrain, select your route through the depression so as to even out the path.

Group Riding

Riding with others is more difficult than you might think, especially if many of the riders are relatively inexperienced. Yet group riding has enormous advantages. The social aspect is one, the mutual encouragement another, as is the fact that a matched group can move faster than any one of the single participants.

But to ride together you have to be predictable. There's no better way to learn it than by joining an established bike club and participating in their group rides. Learn to signal to the others when you are moving out or slowing down, how to point out irregularities in the road and how to tell when it's your time to take the lead or drop back.

The formation that moves fastest is known as the echelon: a bunch of cyclist riding close together, taking turns at the lead. Done correctly, each person only stays in the front for a very short time, so the group is essentially constantly rotating, the last lead rider falling back in line at the end after perhaps ten or twenty pedal strokes in the lead. Stronger riders may take longer and weaker ones shorter turns at the lead, as the group seems to become a single living organism where every member has become part of a greater total. Worth the experience, but impossible to explain in words: join a club to learn to do it right.

4. Using the Gears

Modern bicycles, in the overwhelming majority, are equipped with a sophisticated derailleur system for multiple gearing. To change gear, the chain is shifted onto any chosen combination of chainring and sprocket with the aid of two derailleur mechanisms.

Nowadays, twelve and fourteen speed systems are generally used, although some have only ten speeds and mountain bikes usually have 18 or 21 speed systems. In the case of ten, twelve or fourteen speed set-ups, two chainrings are used in combination with five, six or seven sprockets, respectively. Fifteen, eighteen and 21-speed systems have three chainrings, combined with five, six or seven sprockets, respectively.

The derailleur method of gearing allows minute adaptations of the gear ratio to the cyclist's potential on the one hand, and the terrain, wind resistance and road conditions on the other hand. All that is mere theory, because in reality the majority of people, including most beginning fitness cyclists, plod along in the wrong gear for the work load. Indeed, learning to select the right gear may well provide the biggest single step towards improved cycling speed and endurance. That's the subject of the present chapter.

There is a sound theory behind the principle of gear selection, based on the optimal pedaling rate, which I have covered in several of my other books, such as the *Bicycle Racing Guide*. Interesting though this theory is, one need not wait with applying the technique until it is thoroughly understood. That's why I shall outline the correct use of gearing to the extent you will need it at this point.

The Derailleur System

Fig. 18.18 in Part III of the book shows and names the mechanical components of the derailleur system. The chain runs over two or three chainrings, also referred to as chainwheels, mounted on the RH crank, and any one of five, six or seven sprockets or cogs mounted on a freewheel block at the rear wheel. As long as you are pedaling forward, the chain can be moved from one chainring to the other with the front derailleur or changer, and from one sprocket to another by means of the rear derailleur.

Because the various chainrings and sprockets have different numbers of teeth, the ratio between pedaling speed and the speed with which the rear wheel — and with it the whole bike — is driven changes whenever a different combination is selected. As illustrated in Fig. 4.1, bigger chainrings in the front and smaller sprockets in the rear result in higher gears, smaller chainrings and bigger sprockets give lower gears. Higher gears are selected when cycling is easy, so the available output allows a high riding speed. Select a lower gear when higher resistances must be overcome, such as riding uphill or against a head wind, or when starting off from standstill.

Each derailleur is controlled by means of a shift lever, usually mounted on the frame's down tube. Alternative positions are less convenient on bikes with drop handlebars in the long run. Only mountain bikes, with their flat bars, allow the use of thumb shifters, mounted directly on the handlebars, within easy reach from the hand grips. Make sure derailleurs and shifters match and the former are suitable for the kind of terrain you will

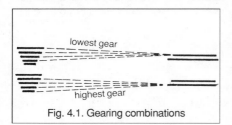

lowest gear

highest gear

Fig. 4.1. Gearing combinations

be encountering. In particular, you need widely spaced gearing if you ride in really hilly terrain a lot.

Most shifts are made with the rear derailleur, while the front changer is primarily used either to find subtle intermediate gears (on the racing bike), or to move from one general range of gears to the other (on the mountain bike).

The rear derailleur is controlled from the RH shifter. To put the chain on a different sprocket in the rear, move the RH shifter, while pedaling forward with reduced force. Pull the lever back to change to a larger sprocket, which results in a lower gear; push it forward to reach a smaller sprocket, resulting in a higher gear.

The LH shift lever controls the front derailleur or changer, which simply shoves the cage through which the chain runs to the left or the right, moving it onto the smaller or the bigger chainring. Pulling the lever back engages the bigger chainring for the higher gear range on most models; pushing it forward engages the smaller chainring, to obtain the lower gearing range.

The Need for Gears

The reason for gearing lies in the possibility it provides to pedal at an efficient rate with comfortable force under a wide range of different conditions and riding speeds. If the combination of chainring and sprocket size were fixed, as it is on the single-speed bicycle, any given pedaling speed invariably corresponds to a certain riding speed. The rear wheel will be turning at a speed that can be simply calculated by multiplying the pedaling rate with the quotient of chainring and sprocket size (expressed in terms of the numbers of teeth):

$$v_{wheel} = v_{pedal} \times T_{front} / T_{rear}$$

where:
v_{wheel} = wheel rotating speed (RPM)
v_{pedal} = pedaling rate (RPM)
T_{front} = number of teeth, chainring

T_{rear} = number of teeth, sprocket

The actual riding speed depends on this wheel rotating speed and the effective wheel diameter. The effective diameter of a nominal 27 inch or 700 mm wheel is about 680 mm. This results in a riding speed in MPH that can be determined by multiplying the wheel speed in RPM by 0.08. These two calculations can be combined to find the riding speed in MPH directly from the pedaling rate and the chainring and sprocket sizes as follows:

$$MPH = 0.08 \times v_{pedal} \times T_{front} / T_{rear}$$

where:
MPH = riding speed in MPH and the other symbols are as defined above. To express riding speed in km/h, use the following formula instead:

$$km/h = 0.125 \times v_{pedal} \times T_{front} / T_{rear}$$

To give an example, assume you are pedaling at a rate of 80 RPM on a bike geared with a 42- tooth chainring and a 21-tooth rear sprocket. Your riding speed, expressed in MPH and km/h respectively, will be:

$$0.08 \times 80 \times 42 / 21 = 13 \text{ MPH}$$

$$0.125 \times 80 \times 42 / 21 = 20 \text{ km/h}$$

Depending on the prevailing terrain conditions, that may be too easy or too hard for optimum endurance performance. If you are riding up a steep incline, this speed may require a very high pedal force, which may well be too exhausting and damaging to muscles, joints and tendons. On a level road the same speed will be reached so easily that you don't feel any significant resistance. All right for cruising, but not if you want the ride to have a training effect.

The derailleur gearing system allows you to choose the combination of chainring and sprocket sizes that enables you to operate effectively at your chosen pedaling speed for optimal performance. You may of course also vary the pedaling rate, which would appear to have the same effect as selecting another gear. Indeed, with any given gear, pedaling slower reduces riding speed and therefore demands less power, whereas a higher pedaling rate increases road speed, requiring more power.

However, power output is not the sole, nor indeed the most important, criterion. Performing work at a given level of power output may tax the body differently depending on the associated forces and speeds of movements. It has been found that to cycle longer distances effectively, without tiring or hurting excessively, the pedal force must be kept down by pedaling at a rate well above what seems natural to the beginning cyclist.

Whereas the beginner tends to plod along at 40—60 RPM, efficient long distance cycling requires pedaling rates of 80 RPM and more, while racers generally pedal even faster. That doesn't come overnight, because the cyclist first has to learn to move his legs that fast, but it is an essential requirement for efficient cycling. Much of your early practice should therefore be aimed at mast-Cadence (see pedaling rate)ering the art of pedaling faster. That must be done in a rather low gear to ensure that training intensity is limited by the factor to be developed, namely muscle speed, rather than by power output or muscle strength.

Gearing Practice

Once you know that high gears mean big chainrings and small sprockets, it's time to get some practice riding in high and low gears. First do it 'dry': the bike supported with the rear wheel off the ground. Turn the cranks by hand and use the shift levers to change up and down, front and rear, until you have developed a good idea of the combinations reached in all conceivable shift lever positions. Listen for rubbing and

crunching noises as you shift, realizing a shift has not been executed properly until the noises have subdued.

Now take to the road. Select a stretch of quiet road, where you can experiment around with your gears without risk of being run into the ground by a closely following vehicle or get in the way of other cyclists. Start off in a low gear and shift the rear derailleur up in steps. Then shift to another chainring and change down through the gears with the rear derailleur — followed by the third chainring if your bike has an 18- or 21-speed system.

Reduce the pedal force, still pedaling forward as you shift. Especially the front derailleur will not shift as smoothly as it did when the cranks were turned by hand. You will notice that the noises become more severe and that some changes just don't take place as you had intended. On a bike without index gearing, you may have to overshift slightly first: push the lever a little beyond the correct position to affect a definite change and then back up until the chain is quiet again. Get a feel for each gear and try to imagine which gear you should select for given conditions. Practice shifting until it goes smoothly and naturally.

Occasionally, it may be necessary to fine-tune the front derailleur position after a change with the rear derailleur. That will be the case when the chain is twisted under an angle that causes it to rub against the side of the front changer. Some people never learn, quite simply because they don't take the trouble to practice consciously. Others take that trouble and learn to shift predictably and smoothly within a week. Half an hour of intensive practice each day during one week, and the continued attention required to do it right during regular riding, is all it takes to become an expert very quickly.

In recent years most manufacturers have introduced indexed derailleur systems with matching freewheel blocks that eliminate the need for fine-tuning. These indexed systems, such as the Shimano SIS and SunTour Accushift, work very well when new. However, a slight misalignment or a little wear can play havoc with the indexing of the various gears. In that case, just move the auxiliary lever to the F-position and use as a non-indexed model until re-adjusted at the bike shop

Gear Designation

Just how high or low any given gear is may be expressed by giving the respective numbers of teeth on chainring and sprocket engaged in the particular gear. However, this is not a very good measure. It may not be immediately clear that a combination designated 42 X 16 has the same effect as one designated 52 X 21, though they really do result in the same ratio, as can be verified mathematically. It will be clear that it becomes nearly impossible to compare gears on bikes with different wheel sizes this way. There must be a better method.

To allow a direct comparison between the gearing effects of different gears and bikes, two methods are in use, referred to as gear number and development, respectively, and illustrated in Fig. 4.2. Gear number is a somewhat archaic method that refers to the equivalent wheel size in inches of a directly driven wheel corresponding to any given combination of wheel size, chainring and sprocket. It is determined by multiplying the quotient of chainring and sprocket sizes with the wheel diameter in inches:

$$gear = D_{wheel} \times T_{front} / T_{rear}$$

where:

$gear$ = gear number in inches
D_{wheel} = wheel diameter in inches
T_{front} = number of teeth, chainring
T_{rear} = number of teeth, sprocket

Returning to the example for a bike with 27-inch wheels, geared with a 42-tooth chainring and a 21-tooth sprocket, the gear number would be:

$$gear = 27 \times 42 / 21 = 54 \text{ in}$$

This is the customary, though rather quaint method used only in the English speaking world to define bicycle gearing. The rest of the world expresses the gear more realistically in terms of development. That is the distance in meters covered by the bike with one crank revolution. Development is calculated as follows:

$$\text{Dev.} = 3.14 \times d_{wheel} \times T_{front} / T_{rear}$$

where:

Dev. = development in meters
d_{wheel} = wheel size in m
T_{front} = number of teeth, chainring
T_{rear} = number of teeth, sprocket

The development for the same example would be:

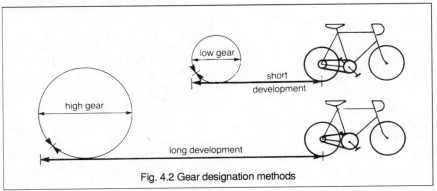

Fig. 4.2 Gear designation methods

Dev. = 3.14 x 0.680 x 42 / 21 = 4.30m

In practice, you are not expected to figure this kind of thing out yourself. Instead you may refer to the tables in the Appendix. Just remember that a high gear is expressed by a high gear number or a long development. For unloaded riding, very low gears in terms of gear number are in the lower thirties (around 2.80—3.20m in terms of development). High gears are those above 90 in (development over 7.20m).

Gear Selection

Possibly the biggest problem for the beginning cyclist is to determine which is the right one out of the bewildering array of available gears. To generalize for most normal cycling conditions, I would say it's whichever gear allows you to maximize your pedaling rate without dimi nishing your capacity to do effective work.

Perhaps you start off with the ability to pedal no faster than 60 RPM. That'll be too low once you have absolved some riding practice, but for now that may be your limit. So the right gear is the one in which you can reach that rate at any time, preferably exceeding it. Count it out with the aid of a wrist watch (or with the pedaling rate device incorporated in

some bicycle computers). If you find yourself pedaling slower, change down into a slightly lower gear, to increase the pedaling rate at the same riding speed. If you're pedaling faster, keep it up until you feel you are indeed spinning too lightly, and only then change into a slightly higher gear to increase road speed at the same pedaling rate.

Gradually, you will develop the ability to pedal faster. As that happens, increase the limiting pedaling rate along with your ability, moving up from 60 to 70, 80 and eventually even higher pedaling rates. When riding with others, don't be guided by their gearing selection, since they may be stronger or weaker, or may have developed their pedaling speed more or less than you have.

It should not take too long before you learn to judge the right gear in advance, without the need to count out the pedal revolutions. You will not only know to change down into a lower gear when the direction of the road changes to expose you to a head wind or when you reach an incline, you will also learn to judge just how far to change down — and up again when the conditions become more favorable. Change gear consciously and frequently in small steps, and you will soon enough master the trick

Derailleur Care and Adjustment

For optimal operation of the derailleur system, several things should be regularly checked and adjusted if necessary. The derailleurs themselves, as well as the chain and the various sprockets, chainrings and control cables, must be kept clean and lightly lubricated. The cables must be just taut when the shift levers are pushed forward and the derailleurs engage the appropriate gear. The tension screw on the shift levers must be kept tightened to give positive shifting without being excessively tight or loose.

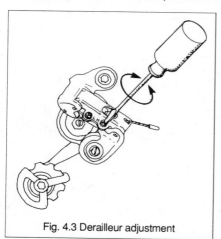

Fig. 4.3 Derailleur adjustment

When the chain gets shifted beyond the biggest or smallest chainring or sprocket, or when certain combinations can not be reached, the derailleurs themselves must be adjusted. For this purpose they are equipped with set-stop screws, which can be adjusted with a small screwdriver, as illustrated in Fig. 4.3. If necessary, place the chain back on the sprocket or chainring, and select a gear that combines a small chainring with a small sprocket. To adjust the front or rear derailleur, proceed as follows:

Adjust Derailleur
1. Establish where the problem lies: front or rear derailleur, shifted too far or not far enough, on the inside or the outside.
2. Determine which of the set-stop screws governs movement limitation in the appropriate direction. On many models these screws are marked with an H and L for high and low gear, respectively. If not, establish yourself which is the appropriate screw by observing what happens at the ends of the screws as you shift towards the extreme gears. The high range set-stop screw is the one towards which an internal protrusion moves as you shift into the highest gear with the appropriate derailleur shift lever.
3. Unscrew the set-stop screw slightly (perhaps half a turn at a time) to increase the range if the extreme gear could not be reached. Tighten it if the chain was shifted beyond that last sprocket.

4. Check all possible combinations to establish whether the system works properly, and fine-tune if necessary.

Derailleur Capacity

Not all derailleurs are capable of handling all possible combinations of gears. As this subject is very complicated, due to the vast array of different makes, models, sizes and combinations of front and rear derailleurs, sprockets and chainrings, it will be impossible to do more than alert you to the problem. Before selecting any uncommon combination, ask in the bike store whether it will work with the equipment you already have on the bike — or intend to install to replace what you have.

In addition to the conventional systems with simple round chainrings, there are some systems on the market that differ. Of the various types that have been introduced from time to time, so far the most prominent is the Shimano Biopace system, installed on virtually all mountain bikes and many fitness machines today. This includes curiously shaped off-round chainrings, available to match the same manufacturer's cranksets. Like all non-standard systems, the Biopace seems to bring an advantage only to those cyclists who have not learned to pedal at a high rate in a relatively low gear. The chainring sizes available for this system are somewhat limited. Nice equipment, but it may be smarter to get used to spinning fast and smoothly, using conventional equipment, selecting your gears consciously.

5. Bicycle Safety

Riding a bicycle is not an entirely risk-less undertaking. Neither are many other pursuits, but what scares off potential cyclists most is probably the danger of being involved in a collision with a motor vehicle. Yes, that chance exists in bicycle riding, as it does when crossing the street in front of your own house. Actually, this is but one of several kinds of possible injury causes in bicycling. You can learn to avoid most of the risks and minimize the impact of these and other injuries and health hazards. These are the subjects of the present chapter and the next one, respectively.

Considering the various risks, ranging from those to your own body and equipment to the harm or loss you may cause others, it may be smart to take out some kind of insurance. Personal liability insurance is perhaps the most important one of these. In addition, you may want to make sure you have adequate health insurance to cover the dangers of the road. This advice may sound exagerated to my British readers, and it is not intended for them: in the US a little accident can cost a fortune in liability claims and health care.

The Risks of Cycling

Quite a lot of research has been done in recent years on the subject of bicycle accidents and injuries. To summarize the available evidence in a nutshell, the majority of bicycle accidents is attributable to a very limited number of typical mistakes, most of which can be either avoided or counteracted by intelligent cycling techniques.

Perhaps the most important lesson to learn from the investigations dealing with the safety of touring cyclists concerns the correlation between risk and trip length. Put simply, the likelihood of getting hurt — be it as a result of a traffic accident or a fall — increases dramatically after a daily distance of 70

miles. Though that applies especially to cyclists carrying luggage and handling difficult terrain, I still advise all beginning riders not to take on those century rides and other monster tours until they are quite experienced and have worked up to that kind of protracted exercise.

Another significant finding is that the more experienced cyclists have markedly fewer accidents, and can go longer distances before being exposed to the greater risk. This is one good argument to try and gain experience and skills as quickly as possible. Following the advice contained in the preceding chapters not only increases the joy, satisfaction and effectiveness of your cycling, it also drastically reduces the risk to which you are exposed.

Traffic Hazards

In the Bikecentennial survey of long distance touring cyclists, only two fatal accidents occurred, which is sad enough. However, fatal accidents are only a small percentage of all injuries, and numerous quite serious accidents do occur. Though the majority of all injured cyclists themselves are largely to blame for their injuries, there always will be some accidents that are directly attributable to bullying and inconsiderate motorists.

Unfortunately, this type of accident forms a high proportion of those that experienced cyclists encounter. These riders have learned to handle their machines rationally and safely in traffic, thus virtually eliminating their risk concerning the more common kinds of accidents to which the incompetent are exposed. Having practically eliminated the latter, they are just as vulnerable to the remaining irrational dangers of the road.

The only defense against inconsiderate road users is not to provoke them. Give in, even if that seems highly unfair. It's an unequal battle and sometimes it's just smarter not to insist on justice. You will encounter fewer of these particular risks if you avoid the kind of situations where they are most likely: Sunday afternoons and late evenings, when many boisterous drunks are on the road. Oddly enough, these accidents are also more likely on relatively lightly travelled roads near smaller towns. Though I realize that busy roads near big cities do not make the ideal cycling environment, you may try to avoid the quiet roads near smaller towns at high-risk times.

Most accidents, of course, are not of this type. They simply happen when two people make a mistake each: one initiates a wrong move, and the other fails to react in such a way that a collision is avoided. Keep that in mind when cycling. Remain alert for the possible mistakes others may make, and try to avoid doing the unexpected or unconsidered yourself as much as humanly possible. Anticipate not only the predictable, but also the unexpected: the motorist looming behind the next corner or intersection, the dog appearing from a driveway, or the bicyclist suddenly crossing your path in the dark without lights.

The latter subject deserves special attention, but the only way to arm yourself is to make sure you do not cycle out after dark without lights yourself, so at least *you* can be seen. Proper lighting on the bike is needed in addition to the curiously ineffective array of reflectors that is increasingly prescribed by law in various countries. The gravest danger of reflectors lies in the inappropriate impression they transmit of your visibility, whereas in reality several of them only make you visible to those who do not endanger you anyway. A bright light in the front and a big rear light or reflector facing back are essential, while all the other goodies won't do a thing that the former wouldn't do more effectively.

Most accidents occur by daylight, even though the relative risk is greater at night. Whether by day or at night, cycle with all your senses alert. In general, ride your bike as you would drive your car, always verifying whether the road ahead of you is clear, and taking particular care to select your path wisely at junctions and intersections. As a relatively slow vehicle, you must look behind you, to ascertain that nobody is following closely, before you move over into another traffic lane or away from your previous path.

Forget anything you ever heard about bikes being different from motor vehicles. As a wheeled vehicle, your bike answers to the same laws of physics as does your car. Adhere to the most basic rules of traffic as you learned them to handle a car as well, and you'll be safe on a bike. No doubt the worst advice ever given to cyclists in many parts of the US is to ride on the side of the road where a pedestrian would go, namely facing traffic. On a bike you *are* the traffic, and you belong on the same side as all other vehicles travelling the same way.

The rules of the road as applied to motor vehicles are based on a logical system that has gradually evolved. This system works the way it does because it is logical and consistent. If it is dangerous for motorists to do certain things, then it will be at least as dangerous on a bike.

Don't hug the curb but claim your place on the road. Your place is about 1.80m (6 ft) to the right of the centerline of the path normally taken by cars on a wide road. Keep at least 90 cm (3 ft) away from the inside edge, even if the road is too narrow to stay clear to the right of the normal path of motor vehicles. Don't dart in and out around parked vehicles and other obstructions along the side of the road.

When making a turn, adhere to the method outlined in Fig. 5.1 (assuming RH traffic). Thus, to go straight at an intersection, make sure you will not be overtaken by vehicles turning right. To turn right, get close to the RH edge. To turn left, choose a path near the center of the road or the middle of a traffic lane marked for that direction well before the actual intersection, after having established that you will not be cutting across the path of vehicles following closely behind.

Excessive attention is often paid to hand signals in traffic education for cyclists. Yes, you should signal your intention before you do things like diverting, turning off or slowing down. That applies particularly when cycling with others in a group, where the first person also should point out and audibly identify obstacles or hazards in the road. But avoid the dangerous habit of assuming a hand signal will ward off danger. Your hand is not a magic wand, and if somebody is following so closely that you can signal to him your intention of turning across his path, you should not do that. Instead, wait until your maneuver does not interfere with traffic following closely behind.

The most feared type of bicycle accident is the one that involves being hit from behind. These accidents do happen, and though there is hardly any defense possible to ward them off, it is worth considering that they are characterized by a number of common factors. They invariably occur on otherwise deserted roads, where the attention of motorist and cyclist alike are at a low, since both feel perfectly secure.

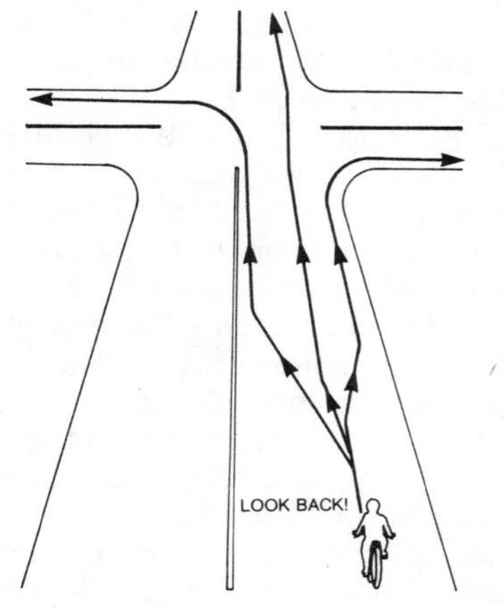

Inconspicuous clothing, a low sun, blinding one or both participants, and a lack of the cyclist's awareness, due to tiredness at the end of a long day, are also common features. It may be smart to increase your conspicuity. Wearing brightly visible colors, such as yellow, pink, orange or bright green, may well help others spot you in time to avoid this type of accident.

Falls and Collisions
Whether or not a motor vehicle is involved, virtually every injury to the cyclist in all falls and collisions results from the impact when the cyclist falls off the bike. He either hits the road surface, an object on or along the road, the colliding vehicle or the bike itself. The same skills necessary to prevent traffic accidents involving cars will keep you from experiencing most of the other types of falls and collisions. Be watchful, consider the effects of your own actions, and use the technical skills described in the preceding chapters to divert when the situation becomes threatening.

Four types of falls and collisions can be distinguished, caused by stopping, diverting, skidding and loss of control, respectively. In the following sections, I shall describe these accidents, each time followed by a few hints about relevant prevention and impact reduction methods.

Stopping Accidents
In a stopping accident, the bicycle runs into an obstacle that halts its progress. Depending on the cyclist's speed, the impact can be very serious. As the bicycle itself is stopped, inertia keeps

LOOK BACK!

Fig. 5.1 Path at junction (RH traffic)

the rider going forward, throwing him against or over the handlebars. The kinetic energy of the moving mass will be dissipated very suddenly, often in an unfortunate location. Your genitals may hit the handlebar stem or your skull may crash ionto something solid.

The way to guard yourself against these accidents is to look and think ahead, so you don't run into any obstacles. If necessary, control your speed to allow handling the unexpected when a potential danger may be looming up behind the next corner. Learn to apply the diverting technique described in Chapter 3. The way to minimize the impact of the most serious form of stopping accident, which will be discussed more fully in Chapter 6, is by wearing an energy absorbing helmet.

Diverting Accidents

A diverting type accident occurs when the front wheel is pushed sideways by an external force, while the rider is not leaning in the same direction to regain balance. Typical causes are railway tracks, cracks in the road surface, the edge of the road, but also touching another rider's rear wheel with your front wheel. The effect is that you fall sideways and hit the road or some obstacle by the side of the road. Depending how unexpectedly it happened, you may be able to reduce the effect of the fall by stretching out an arm, which seems to be an automatic reflex in this situation.

Characteristic injuries range from abrasions and lacerations of the hands and the sides of arms and legs to bruised hips and sprained or broken wrists. More serious cases, usually incurred at higher speeds, may involve broken collarbones and injuries to the face or the side of the skull. The impact of the lesser injuries can be minimized by wearing padded gloves and double layers of clothing with long sleeves and legs. Wearing a helmet will minimize damage to the side of the head, espe-

cially at elevated speeds.

Diverting accidents can often be avoided if the cyclist is both careful and alert. Keep an eye out for the typical danger situations. Don't overlap wheels with other riders, don't approach surface ridges under a shallow angle. A last second diversion can often be made along the lines of the diverting technique described in Chapter 3. In the case of a ridge in the road surface, use the technique of sideways jumping, also de scribed there. When your front wheel touches the rear wheel of another rider, or if your handlebars are pushed over by an outside force, you may sometimes save the day if you react by immediately leaning in the direction into which you were diverted, and then steer to regain control.

Skidding Accidents

When the bicycle keeps going or goes in an unintended direction, despite your efforts to brake or steer, it will be due to skidding between the tires and the road surface. This kind of thing happens more frequently when the road is slick on account of moisture, frost, loose sand or fallen leaves. Especially under these conditions, sudden diversions or movements, hard braking and excessive lean when cornering may all cause skidding either forward or sideways.

Skidding accidents often also cause the cyclist to fall sideways, resulting in abrasions, lacerations or more rarely fractures. Avoid them by checking the road surface ahead and avoiding sudden steering or braking maneuvers and excessive leaning in curves. Cross slick patches, ranging from wet or greasy as- phalt to railway tracks, from sand or leaves on the road to the white lines used as road markings, with the bicycle upright. Achieve that by carrying out the requisite steering and balancing actions *before* you reach such danger spots.

If you can not avoid it, once you feel you are entering a skid, try to move your weight towards the back of the bike as much as possible, sliding back on the saddle and stretching the arms. Follow the bike, rather than trying to force it back. Finally, don't do what seems an obvious reaction to the less experienced, namely getting off the saddle to straddle the top tube with one leg dangling.

Loss of Control Accidents

At higher speeds, especially in a steep descent, loss of control accidents sometimes occur. In this case, you just can't steer the bike the way you intend to go. This happens when you find yourself having to steer in one direction at a time when you are leaning the other way, or when speed control braking initiates unexpected oscillations. Often this situation develops into a collision or a fall along the lines of either one of the accident types described above.

Prevention is only possible with experience: don't go faster than the speed at which you feel in control. The more you ride under various conditions, the more you will develop a feel for what is a safe speed, when to brake and how to steer to maintain control over the bike. Once the situation sets in, try to keep your cool. Don't panic. Follow the bike, rather than forcing it over. The worst thing you can do is to tense up and get off the saddle. Stay in touch with handlebars, seat and pedals, and steer in the direction of your lean. This way, you may well get out of it without falling or colliding, though your nerves may have suffered.

6. Bicycling Health

Since the most common health aspect of cycling — namely the pursuit of fitness — is adequately treated elsewhere in this book, this chapter is devoted to some of the other aspects of physical well being. Here, the other side of the safety coin will be discussed: what to do to treat or avoid injuries or other health hazards associated with cycling. Most of these things are not particularly dangerous, but incorrect treatment can aggravate things, and this chapter will help you minimize the risks.

Treating Abrasions

Abrasions, referred to in club cycling circles as road rash, are the most common cycling injury resulting from any kind of fall. They usually heal relatively fast, though they can be quite painful. Wash out the wound with water and soap, and remove any particles of road dirt to prevent infection. There may be a risk of tetanus if the wound draws blood. If you have been immunized against tetanus, get a tetanus shot within 24 hours only if the last one was more than two years ago.

If you have never been immunized before, get a full immunization, consisting of two shot within 24 hours, followed by two more after two weeks and six months, respectively. Apply a dressing only if the location is covered by clothing, since the wound will heal faster when exposed to the air. Avoid the formation of a scab by treating the wound with an antibiotic salve. See a doctor if any signs of infection occur, such as swelling, itching or fever.

Sprained Limbs

In case of a fall, your tendency to stick out an arm to break the impact may result in a sprained or even a fractured wrist. In other accident situations this can also happen to the knee or the ankle. Spraining is really nothing but damage to the ligaments that surround and hold the various parts of a joint together. Typical symptoms are a local sensation of heat, itching and swelling.

Whenever possible, keep the area cold with an ice bag. If you feel a stinging pain or if fever develops, get medical advice, because it may actually be a fracture that was at first incorrectly diagnosed as a sprain. This may be the case when the fracture takes the form of a simple 'clean' crack without superficially visible deformation of the bone.

Fractures

Typical cycling fractures are those of the wrist and the collarbone, both caused when falling: the one when extending the arm to brake the fall, the other when you don't have time to do that. You or medical personnel may not at first notice a clean fracture as described above: there may be one without any outward sign.

If there is a stinging pain when the part is moved or touched, I suggest you get an X-ray to make sure, even if a fracture is not immediately obvious. You'll need medical help to set and bandage the fractured location, and you must give up cycling (except perhaps on the windload simulator or home trainer, spinning lightly if you are really hooked on cycling) until it is healed, which will take about five weeks. Sad if that happens during the preparation for an important event, but better than continuing in agony.

Head Injuries

If you fall on your head in any kind of accident, the impact may smash the brain against the inside of the skull, followed by the reverse action as it bounces back. The human brain can usually withstand this kind of treatment without lasting damage if the resulting deceleration does not exceed 300G, or about $3000m/sec^2$. Look at it this way: the head probably falls to the ground from a height of 1.5m (5 ft). This results in a speed of 5m/sec^2 at the time of impact. To keep the deceleration down below 3000m/sec, this speed must be reduced to zero in no less than 0.002 sec.

Neither your skull, nor the object with which you collide is likely to deform gradually enough to achieve even that kind of deceleration. That's why energy absorbing helmets with thick crushable foam shells were developed. Neither flexible nor hard materials will do the trick by themselves. It's not a bad idea to have a hard outer shell cover to distribute the load of a point impact, and it is nice to get some comfort inside from a soft flexible liner, but the crushing of about $^3/4$ inch of seemingly brittle foam is essential to absorb the shock. The minimum requirement for a safe helmet is the American standard ANSI Z-90.4.

Other Health Problems

The remaining part of this chapter will be devoted to the health hazards of cycling that have nothing to do with falling off the bike. We will look at the most common complaints and discuss some methods of prevention, as well as possible cures. This brief description can not cover the entire field. Nor should most of the issues discussed here be generalized too lightly. The same symptoms may have different causes in different cases; conversely, the same cure may not work for two superficially similar problems. Yet in most cases the following remarks will apply.

Saddle Sores

Though beginning bicyclists may at first feel uncomfortable on the bike seat, they have no idea what kind of agony real seat problems can bring. In cycling for fitness, much more than in racing, you have the opportunity to avoid the most serious seat problems by taking a break from cycling when symptoms start to develop. Racers and other long-dis-

tance riders often have a much harder time at it. What happens during the many hours in the saddle is that the combined effect of perspiration, pressure and chafing causes cracks in the skin where dirt and bacteria can enter. The result can be anything from a mild inflammation to the most painful boils.

There is of course little chance of these things healing as long as you continue riding vigorously. As soon as any pressure is applied, when you sit on a bike seat, things will get worse. Prevention and early relief are the methods to combat saddle sores. The clue to both is hygiene. Wash and dry both your crotch and your cycling shorts after every day's ride. Many bicyclists also treat the affected area with rubbing alcohol, which both disinfects and increases the skin's resistance to chafing, or with talcum powder, which prevents further damage.

You'll need at least two pairs of shorts, certainly if you ever ride two days in a row, so you can always rely on a clean, dry pair when you go out. Wash them out, taking particular care to get the chamois clean, and hang them out to dry thoroughly, preferably outside, where the sun's ultraviolet rays may act to kill any remaining bacteria. Treat the chamois with either talcum powder or a special treatment for that purpose. I prefer to use a water soluble cream, such as Noxema, since it is easiest to wash out.

The quality of your saddle and your riding position may also affect the development of crotch problems. If early symptoms appear in the form of redness or soreness, consider getting a softer saddle, sitting further to the back of your saddle, or lowering the handlebars a little to reduce the pressure on the seat. If the problem gets out of hand, take a rest from cycling until the sores have fully healed.

While your sore spots are healing, continue your fitness program running, stretching and doing calisthenics.

Knee Problems

Because the cycling movement does not apply the high impacting shock loads on the legs that are associated with running, it's surprising that knee problems are so prevalent. They are mainly concentrated with two groups of cyclists: beginners and very strong, muscular riders. In both cases, the cause seems to be pushing too high a gear. This places excessive forces on the knee joint, resulting in damage to the membranes that separate the moving portions of the joint and the ligaments holding the bits and pieces together. In cold weather the problems get aggravated, so it will be wise to wear long pants whenever the temperature is below 18°C (65°F), especially if fast descents are involved.

Prevent excessive forces on the knee joint by gearing so low that you can spin lightly under all conditions, avoiding especially climbing in the saddle with pedaling speeds below 60 RPM. Equip your bicycle with the kind of gear ratios that allow you to do that, and choose a lower gear whenever necessary. Once the problem has developed, either giving up cycling or riding loosely in low gears will aid the healing process. I suggest you continue cycling in very low gears, spinning freely. That will probably prepare you to get back into shape, while forcing you to avoid the high gears that caused the problem in the first place.

Tendinitis

This is an infection of the Achilles tendon, which attaches the big muscle of the lower leg, the gastrocnemius, to the heel bone. It is an important tendon in cycling, since the pedaling force can not be applied to the foot without it. It sometimes gets damaged or torn under the same kind of conditions as described above for knee injuries: cycling with too much force in too high a gear. The problem is aggravated by low temperatures, which explains why it generally develops in the early season.

To avoid tendinitis, wear long woollen socks whenever the temperature is below 18°C (65°F). It may also help to wear shoes that come up quite high, maximizing the support they provide. Get used to riding with a supple movement in a low gear, which seems to be the clue to preventing many cycling complaints. Healing requires rest, followed by a return to cycling with minimum pedal force in a low gear.

Numbness

Especially beginning cyclists, not yet used to riding longer distances, sometimes develop a loss of feeling in certain areas of contact with the bike. The most typical location is the hands, but it also occurs in the feet and the crotch. This is caused by excessive and unvaried prolonged pressure on the nerves and blood vessels. The effects are usually relieved with rest, though they have at times been felt for several days.

Once the problem develops, get relief by changing your position frequently, moving the hands from one part of the handlebars to another, or moving from one area of the seat to another if the crotch is affected. To prevent the numbness in the various locations, use well padded gloves, foam handlebar sleeves, a soft saddle in a slightly higher position, or thick soled shoes with cushioned inner soles, laced loosely at the bottom but tightly higher up, depending on the location of the numbness.

Back Ache

Many riders complain of aches in the back, the lower neck and the shoulders, especially early in the season. These are probably attributable to insufficient training of the muscles in those locations. It is largely the result of unfamiliar isometric muscle work, keeping still in a forward bent position. This condition may also be partly caused or aggravated by low temperatures, so it is wise to wear warm bicycle clothing in cool weather.

To avoid the early-season reconditioning complaints, the best remedy is not to interrupt cycling in winter. Even two longer rides a week at a moderate pace, or extended use of a home trainer with a proper low riding position, will do the trick. Alternately, you may start off in the new season with a slightly higher handlebar position and once more a low gear. Sleeping on a firm mattress and keeping warm also seems to either help alleviate or prevent the problem.

Sinus and Bronchial Complaints

Especially in the cooler periods, many cyclists develop breathing problems, originating either in the sinuses or the bronchi. The same may happen when a rider used to cycling at sea level gets into the mountains, where the cold air in a fast descent can be very unsettling. It is generally attributable to undercooling, the only solution being to dress warmer and to cycle slowly enough to allow breathing through the nose.

After a demanding climb in cooler weather, do not strip off warm clothing, open your shirt or drink excessive quantities of cold liquids, even if you sweat profusely. All these things cause more rapid cooling than your body may be able to handle. You will cool off gradually and without impairing your health if you merely reduce your output and allow the sweat to evaporate through the fibers of your clothing, especially if it contains a high percentage of wool.

Sun Burn

When cycling, you will be exposed to the sun for many hours at a stretch. Unless you have a naturally high resistance to ultra violet light, exposed parts of the body are likely to suffer sun burn. To prevent it, use a sun tan lotion with a protection factor of 15. This means that only one fifteenth of the ultra violet rays reach the skin. Even more effective is zinc oxide based protection, applied in selected locations such as the nose the ears and the neck.

Sun burn is just that: a burn, and that means it should be treated like any other burn. Cold water and perhaps a light dressing such as baby oil are all you can do, apart from waiting for it to heal. In really severe cases, sun burn can be serious enough to justify professional medical care. There are substances that suppress the pain, but there is little chance of healing a burn with any kind of treatment.

Overtraining

Though this phenomenon is more commonly associated with the pursuit of bicycle racing, it can occur amongst ambitious fitness bicyclists as well. While it is not usually recognized as a cycling injury, it should be treated as one. There are certain symptoms associated with overtraining and there are real hazards in ignoring these. It is simply a matter of having pushed your body beyond its present limits by cycling too far too fast.

The symptoms include excessive nervousness, tension and perspiration, as well as a rapid pulse. To overcome the problem, take it easy for one week, and then gradually increase the workload.

The morning pulse is a convenient indicator. If it increases more than it usually does between lying in bed and just after getting up, you'd better take it easy for a couple of days. Perhaps equally useful is to ask yourself how you are feeling in general. If you have difficulty sleeping and tire more than usual, if you feel listless, have a poor appetite, perspire more than usual or feel unjustified anxiety, it will be time to suspect overtraining. See a doctor if a few days' relative rest does not solve the problem.

Part II – Training For Fitness

7. What Makes the Bicycle Go?

It is easier to reach an optimal cycling performance if one understands which factors affect the bicycle's speed. The things that make it go, and those that limit its performance, can and should be comprehended if you want to get the most out of the machine. That will be the subject of the present chapter.

Cycling versus Running

Cycling is more efficient than walking and running. With the same physical output necessary to walk at 5km/h (3 mph), the cyclist proceeds four times as fast. A comparison of athletic performance will demonstrate that at maximum output levels, the cyclist invariably goes at about twice the runner's speed. The difference lies in the energy required to lift the body several inches with every step the walker takes (see Fig. 7.1). This energy, which can be computed by multiplying the lifting height by the number of steps, is lost to forward motion in walking.

When cycling, the athlete's body remains at the same height, and in consequence essentially all energy used is recovered in forward motion. Even if the cyclist gets out of the saddle, his weight subsequently works via the bicycle's drive-train to bring him forward. It is as though the walker could roll down a little ramp from the high point of each step he took. But cycling is even more effective, since the speed remains more constant than it does when walking. The only cyclic acceleration and deceleration is that of the rider's legs, not the much greater mass of the entire body, as is the case for the walker.

Just the same, cycling is no perpetuum mobile, because there are certain resistances to overcome when riding the bicycle. On a level road these losses are attributable primarily to wheel rolling resistance, air (or wind) resistance and friction. In addition, power will be required to get up to speed, and the gravitational effect must be overcome

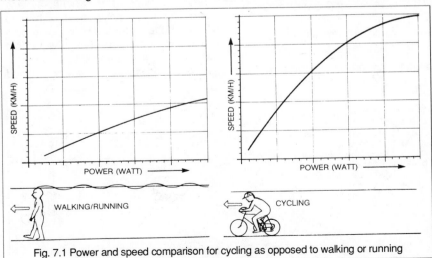

Fig. 7.1 Power and speed comparison for cycling as opposed to walking or running

on inclines. Because the latter form is a useful device to illustrate the other losses, we'll treat it first.

The Effect of Gravity

Consider the situation depicted in Fig. 7.2. The cyclist must overcome gravity over a vertical distance of 1000m (approx. 3500 ft), cycling up a steeply inclined road. Compared to the effect of gravity, all other resistances are of a minor nature under these circumstances (low speed, high output). So, in fact it amounts to the situation depicted as the cyclist's vision: pulling up a heavy weight over a given distance. The distance is the vertical difference that must be overcome, 1000m in this case. The weight equals that of bike and rider. I have assumed a weight of 750N (N stands for Newton, the scientific unit for force; in non-scientific units the equivalent would be approx. 170 lbs).

The total amount of work (or energy, which is another name for the same concept) required to overcome the effect of gravity can be calculated as the product of height and weight force:

$$W = S \times F$$

where:
W = work in Nm (Newton-meter) or J (Joule — equivalent to Nm)
S = vertical distance in m
F = weight force in N

In the illustrated situation that will be:

$$W = 1000m \times 750N = 750{,}000Nm$$

At whatever speed you climb that hill, the total amount of work required will always be the same. The difference between going faster or slower affects not the work, but the power, which can be considered the intensity of work in terms of time. Power is calculated as the quotient of work divided by time:

$$P_i = F / t$$

where:
P_i = power required to overcome gradient in Nm/sec or watt (equivalent units)
F = weight force (or weight) in N
t = time in sec

To do the given amount of work in 30 min (or 1800 sec) takes:

$$P_i = 750{,}000J / 1800 \text{ sec} = 420 \text{ watt}$$

Done in half the time, the climb will require twice the power: 840 watt (about 1.12 hp) in the present example.

The foregoing calculations apply solely to the gravitational effect. In reality, more work and power will be required in each instance, since the overall efficiency is reduced by the other losses. Generally, climbing does not take place on such a steep incline as used here to illustrate the effect of gravity. When the incline is less steep, the gravity effect will become less dominant compared to the other resistances, as will be clarified

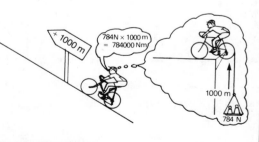

The work required to overcome gravity when riding up a steep incline amounts to the same as would be needed to pull the weight of bike and rider up over the vertical distance equivalent to the height of the hill.

Fig. 7.2 Effect of hill climbing

below in the section *Total Resistance, Speed and Power*.

It may be useful to look at the gravitational effect in terms of the required power as a function of the steepness of the incline (or the power bonus received on a decline, which will speed you up when going downhill). This may be done with the aid of the following formulas for power and resistance force respectively, and as illustrated in Fig. 7.3:

$$P_i = R_i \times v$$
$$R_i = 100 \times i \times F$$

where:

P_i = power required to overcome gravitational force on incline

R_i = effective gravitational resistance in N on given incline

v = riding speed in m/sec

i = gradient or incline in percent (negative value for downslope)

F = total weight of bicycle and rider in N

Other Resistances

In real life, the effect of gravity is only significant for uphill stretches. However, it is one good way to explain the effect of various resistances when cycling. To list them all, the resistances of cycling are:

- Gravitational resistance (depending on steepness);
- Rolling resistance of the tires on the road (depending on tire pressure and deformation);
- Air resistance (depending on frontal area, aerodynamic qualities of bike, components and cycling dress, and highly dependent on riding speed);
- Mechanical friction in the transmission and other moving parts (depen
ding on quality and state of lubrication)
- Acceleration resistance (depending on the rate of speed increase and the mass of bike and rider, particularly of moving parts).

The individual resistances can be calculated similarly. Thus the power required to propel the bicycle under given circumstances and a given speed can also be calculated, simply by multiplying the resistance with the relevant speed.

Total Resistance, Speed and Power

In the preceding section, we have mentioned each of the various resistances that must be overcome. Now it is time to

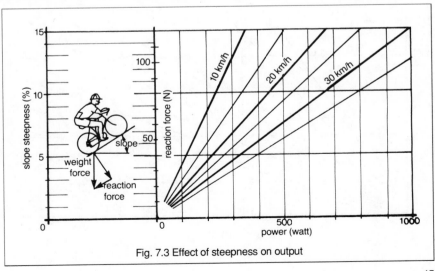

Fig. 7.3 Effect of steepness on output

add them together in order to determine just how much power is required to propel the bicycle at a certain speed, or conversely which speed will be reached with a given power output under various conditions.

I shall not bore you with any more details, instead just presenting the summary of these calculations in the form of a number of graphs, Fig. 7.4, 7.5 and 7.6, representing the power required on a level road, the additional power required for hill climbing and the additional power required to accelerate, respectively. In formula form, the following totals apply:

$$P = (F_i + F_r + F_d + m\,a)\,v\,/\,\mu$$

where:

P = total required power in watt to propel the bike at a given speed

v = speed in m/sec

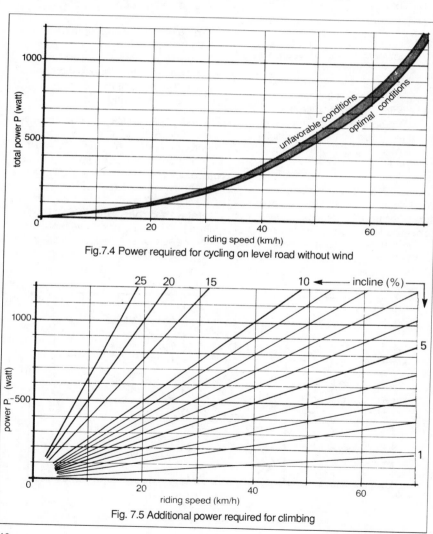

Fig.7.4 Power required for cycling on level road without wind

Fig. 7.5 Additional power required for climbing

μ   =   εφφιχιενχψ
F_i =   esistance force due to incline in N
F_r =   rolling resistance force in N
F_d =   air drag resistance force in N
m   =   mass of bike and rider in kg
         (including a factor doubling the
         wheel mass for greater accuracy
a   =   acceleration in m/sec^2

Conclusions

If you learn nothing else from this dis-
course, just note that cycling is not a
mystical but a physical science: you get
out what you put in and the required
power or the resulting speed can be calculated by those who are into these

things.

When someone tries to convince you
that a bike has mysterious climbing or
accelerating powers, ask for the facts:
how heavy is the bike and its moving
parts, what is the rolling resistance of the
tires used, and where does it differ from
other bikes.

Ninety-nine times out of a hundred,
someone is trying to sell you a bill of
goods: there are no mysterious qualities
in one bike that are not in any other
machine of the same weight and with
similar tires at the same speed. In that
case, you'll have to put in the same effort to propel the one as the other.

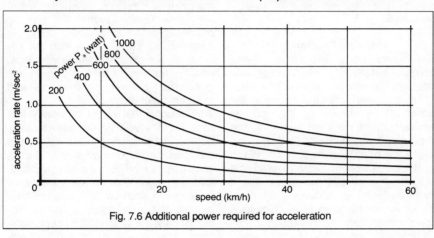

Fig. 7.6 Additional power required for acceleration

8. What Makes the Cyclist Go?

In the present chapter we shall take a close look at the cyclist as the motor that must produce the power to overcome the various resistances described in Chapter 7. First we shall concentrate on the total power trained and untrained cyclists have to offer under various circumstances. In the next section we'll compare available power with the power required to reach a particular speed, to establish which speeds can be attained under any given set of conditions. The detailed processes by which power is generated and work is performed by the cyclist's muscles will be explained in Chapter 9.

Physical Efficiency

The human body takes in food and oxygen, converts it into energy and releases the waste products. The energy intake over a longer period can be established by counting the energy equivalency of the food intake. In the short run this figure is of little use, because the body doesn't burn off all the food it takes in right away. Instead, the oxygen intake can be used as a measure for the work done, since there is a known relationship between oxygen consumption and energy output.

Generally, about 75% of all the energy is turned into heat, whereas about 25% is converted into mechanical work. To put it another way, the human body's mechanical efficiency is 0.25. Actually, that is better than it may seem at first sight, since this is a ratio reached or exceeded only by the most modern industrial power plants, while your car engine and most steam turbines are quite a bit less efficient.

The efficiency is of some importance to our investigation of the cyclist's performance. It is customary in books covering this subject of research to refer to laboratory tests in which the cyclist's power output level have been measured on a bicycle ergometer. Older tests of this type have left much to be desired. Some such supposedly scientific work has been claimed to demonstrate clearly that cycling at any speed suitable for fitness cycling would be impossible — or at least undesirable.

The problem with many older tests is that the researchers had concentrated too much on efficiency. They didn't understand the fact that the bicyclist isn't necessarily riding his bicycle in an attempt to conserve oxygen and calories. By concentrating solely on establishing the point of maximum efficiency, these researchers were ignoring the cyclist's desire to proceed and his ability to deliver more power, even if at the expense of a slight decrease in efficiency, which is nothing more than an increase in the ratio between heat energy and mechanical energy.

Measuring the body's efficiency has its uses in the field of bicycle physiology. But not for predicting what will be the best pedaling rate or what would be a good output level during a race. Instead, efficiency comparisons are suitable for determining such variables as the best posture and pedaling style. The recommendations for criteria like seat height, body angle and crank length in this book are based on such tests. For example, if at all output levels one seat height or crank length is associated with greater efficiency, that one should be used for that rider.

Measuring Power and Energy

Though in recent years researchers who are adequately familiar with bicycle racing have been conducting laboratory tests that go well beyond mere comparisons of physical efficiency, my approach is slightly different again. I refer to the large body of reliable data that is available from real-world cycling. Combining the calculations in the preceding chapter with the results from actual time trials over various distances provides data that are both reliable and supremely relevant to the subject of bicycling for fitness. Wherever I have based my discussion in this and the preceding chapter on published laboratory data, I have verified the data's practical validity by comparing it with the undeniable facts of the real cycling world.

The total amount of energy delivered during a given period can be estimated by such a combination of theoretical and empirical work. This is done most accurately by comparing the total mileage traveled with the speed and other factors influencing the power for each section of the course. A simple substitute is to merely base the estimate on the total time and the average speed, either considering a multiplier factor for terrain conditions or adding the calculated energy required to overcome given climbs or head winds.

To establish just how much power a particular rider — you, for instance— can generate on a bicycle, one only has to compare the required time for a given distance with the graphs from the preceding chapter, either in real life or on such a handy ergometer device as the Cat-Eye CycloSimulator, with its built-in output measuring device.

For real life testing by riding a bike, two situations seem most suitable: a prolonged time trial and a steep hill climb. A long time trial on a level road gives a good measure of the power that can be produced during the time required to complete it and can be repeated for various distances. The hill climbing situation requires the cyclist to ride up a short steep incline (10% or more) with a known elevation gain, to establish maximum power available during a short period by comparing the average speed achieved with graph 7.5. Repeating the same test from time to time, preferably riding a similar, but not the same, stretch of road, will give a good check on training progress.

Available Power

The power that an athlete has available to propel his bicycle eventually determines the speed at which he can ride or the rate at which he can accelerate to reach a higher speed. Different people of course have widely varying physiques, and consequently can produce entirely different power outputs. Some of this difference is genetically deter-

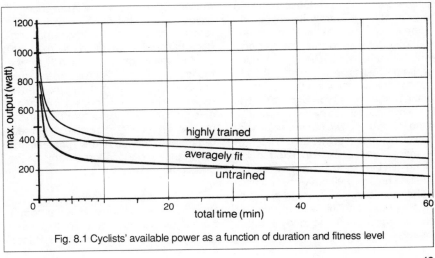

Fig. 8.1 Cyclists' available power as a function of duration and fitness level

mined, but a significant portion is the direct result of training. Thus there is probably enough room for improvement, even if you should not be so genetically endowed as to be a predestined champion.

Fig. 8.1 shows typical (though by no means universally representative) performance curves that relate the maximum power output to the time duration for which each power level can be maintained. These curves are for three types of cyclists: a highly trained racer, a reasonably fit cyclist, and an untrained rider. All three are familiar enough with cycling to allow the use of these curves to determine their actual performance potential (a non-cyclist, tested the same way, would deliver even less power than the untrained rider, since his cycling motion is not yet smooth and natural).

Note that these curves do not represent continuous power at the levels shown: each power output level on the curve can only be maintained during the corresponding time, followed by rest. In other words, if the 400 watt output is required of the trained racer for 30 min, this must be a pretty constant output from beginning to end, and followed by rest. If, on the other hand, one of the higher values in the LH portion of the curve are expended first, this same output cannot be delivered any more.

The most important things to observe on these curves are their relative position and their shape. Clearly, the curve for the trained racer lies higher than for the less trained cyclist, while the curve for the untrained person lies even lower. The aim of the fitness cyclist is to first get to the lower of the two curves shown and then climb up to a point between the two — unless you decide to expand into racing at a later date, when you won't be satisfied until you hit the upper curve.

The racer can deliver more power for any time duration. This is the primary effect of training on the body's output potential. Although an inherently strong

untrained individual may deliver more power than an inherently weaker person, the effect of proper training will be to raise the curve for any one athlete.

Long Term and Short Term Power

Let us now consider the shape of these curves. You will notice that power decreases with time, but by no means linearly: at first it drops off very steeply, and quite soon becomes much less steep. The most significant aspect is the pronounced difference between very short duration and long duration power. For very short periods, an enormous power output can be delivered — well over 750 watt (1 hp). As the time over which the effort must be maintained increases, the power drops off rapidly. At one or two minutes the curves bend quite abruptly and decline much less steeply from there on. In the next section we'll see why this is so.

The distinct difference between the short duration high power and long duration low power output portions of the curves can be attributed to the significance of anaerobic work where short duration high power output is delivered. The terms aerobic and anaerobic have become such buzz-words, that it may seem in order to clarify their meaning. Aerobic means in the presence of oxygen, anaerobic without oxygen, here referring to the mechanisms that produce the ATP (adenosine triphosphate) in the mitochondria, which are the muscle's power cells. ATP is the substance that generates the muscle energy, as it is itself broken down. The available muscle energy is proportional to the number of ATP molecules formed, regardless whether the process by which that is done is the aerobic or the anaerobic pathway.

Aerobic Power

Aerobic power generation is the body's normal operating mode. In this case glucose molecules from the blood stream are broken down completely to form 38 ATP molecules each, as they are burned with the oxygen (hence the term aerobic) that is also carried in the blood. This is the most efficient way of producing energy; besides, it can be called a 'clean process', producing minimal waste to load the blood stream, which means less fatigue. However, it is relatively slow and limited by the body's capacity to carry oxygen to the muscle's mitochondria. The duration over which aerobic power may be given off relatively painlessly is limited by the amount of glucose stored in the blood.

Within the limits of strength of the muscles, the maximum aerobic power (i.e. the intensity of aerobic work performed in a certain time period) is limited by the cardio-respiratory capacity. That is the amount of oxygen lungs and heart can deliver via the blood stream to the muscles. The cardio-respiratory capacity is generally expressed in terms of $\dot{V}_{O2max}$. That is the maximum volume of oxygen related to total body weight that is absorbed per minute. Typical values range from 30ml/kg for an untrained healthy person to 80ml/kg for world class road racers. Though training can increase it quite a bit, as the heart muscle is strengthened, some people just naturally have a bigger capacity than others, which makes them potentially more successful aerobic performers: stronger long distance cyclists.

An individual rider's current $\dot{V}_{O2max}$ may be established experimentally. Though it can be done most accurately in a sports or work physiology lab, it is possible to estimate your own $\dot{V}_{O2max}$ with the aid of a windload simulator or a bicycle ergometer. The instruction manuals for most of these machines include detailed descriptions for estimating $\dot{V}_{O2max}$ and various other fitness tests. Such tests will be accurate to within 10%, except perhaps for very highly trained endurance athletes (who probably have easier access to more sophisticated testing techniques anyway). I recommend repeating the test to estimate $\dot{V}_{O2max}$ twice a year. Comparing results of subsequent tests allows you to establish whether your $\dot{V}_{O2max}$ is still increasing. It will continue to increase as long as you are training effectively and have not reached your absolute maximum yet.

Even amongst advanced fitness cyclists and bicycle racers there are wide differences in $\dot{V}_{O2max}$. Those in the higher categories of road racing almost all have high capacities, suggesting perhaps that there is little hope for more modestly endowed athletes. However, even in road racing people with modest $\dot{V}_{O2max}$ but good sprinting power may keep up with the top in a close pack, eventually beating them in the sprint. Amongst track sprinters and other short-distance specialists, high $\dot{V}_{O2max}$ levels are the exception, rather than the rule, since their disciplines depend more on anaerobic power than on the long term aerobic power supply.

Anaerobic Power

The anaerobic mode is strongly activated when much higher output levels are required. Two metabolic systems constitute anaerobic power generation, referred to as ATP-CP and lactic acid systems, respectively. In the ATP-CP, or high energy phosphates mechanism, creatine phosphate (CP) is the source of ATP in a single enzyme reaction.

The ATP-CP system operates extremely fast. It is limited by the amount of CP stored in the muscle tissue, and depends on the presence of favorable conditions for the enzyme reaction. It can provide short duration maximum energy bursts of up to about 15 seconds. In practice, this system is more important than meets the eye, since it is called upon just a little each time muscle forces exceed the low levels that can be permanently supported. That can be during the peak portion of every pedal stroke, e.g. while climbing or accelerating. The ATP and CP stores in the muscle, though depleted within 15 seconds of maximum output, are recovered relatively fast, namely within about three minutes.

The other kind of anaerobic power is generated in what is referred to as the lactic acid system, and can supply energy for up to about two minutes at peak performance. It leads to a degree of depletion from which the body takes a long time to recover, and should therefore not be used, except in short duration events or near the end of a ride.

In this system, a reaction called glycolysis takes place. In glycolysis, sugars (both the glucose from the blood and the glycogen stored in the muscle and liver tissue) are broken down without oxygen (hence the term anaerobic) to form ATP. In this process, an excess of lactic acid is formed. Lactic acid is also formed in other metabolic processes. However, whereas the small quantity resulting from aerobic work is immediately reconverted in aerobic work, the excess remains to be oxidized in the case of anaerobic work. This is the reason for the oxygen debt (heavy breathing, and sometimes dizziness after the work is done) that often results from anaerobic work.

The lactic acid process is fast and powerful, but wasteful in terms of energy efficiency. Each glucose molecule produces only two ATP molecules, as compared to 38 ATP molecules in the aerobic process. If all your power were to be provided this way, a given food intake would only allow you to cycle perhaps 10 miles a day. However, so many more ATP molecules can be formed within a given (brief) time, that high output levels are possible. The power limitation — apart from the muscle's strength — lies in the conditions favorable to the enzyme reaction involved. These are largely influenced by specific training methods that stress the system and require correct food and favorable temperature conditions. The time during which this energy may be used is limited by the amount of stored sugars and the accumulation of lactic acid. It is assumed that training methods that frequently call on this metabolism may stimulate the removal of lactic acid, thus perhaps leading to an increase of time during which the powerful lactic acid system may be relied on.

Unlike its aerobic counterpart, the level of anaerobic power cannot be easily established riding a bicycle by the amateur researcher, since too many other variables affect the time in a furious sprint. Instead, you may use a simple variant of the method employed in many laboratories to estimate this characteristic. Run up a flight of stairs as fast as you can, three steps at a time, while letting someone record the time, accurate to 0.1 sec, required to gain a certain height. Then calculate the maximum power for that time from the following formula:

$$P = h \times F / t$$

where:

P = power in watt
F = weight in Newton (obtain by multiplying weight in lbs by 4.7 or kg by 9.8)
t = time in seconds

To put it all into some perspective, you may be interested to know what a really good sprinter can deliver anaerobically. A fast sprint of 200 m is ridden in approx. 10 sec, and that corresponds to a power output of more than 1000 watt or 1.4 hp.

Anaerobic Threshold

An athlete's anaerobic threshold is thought of as the level of power beyond which the anaerobic high energy phosphate and lactic acid systems are activated to a significant extent. This is the level at which the available oxygen is no longer adequate to break down and absorb the lactic acid resulting from anaerobic work. I find it dangerous to think of this point as a distinct output level. Even if it is, there remains the problem of establishing just where it lies. My experience, shared by at least some scientists, is that this supposed threshold may be at one level today and at another tomorrow, even for the same rider. And as for establishing it, I am not satisfied with any conventional objective method.

Essentially, aerobic power is delivered whenever work is done. But so is anaerobic power: very little at low, very much at high output levels. The ATP-CP system is called upon for both short bursts of power and for the brief peak muscle forces. When power demands increase beyond the maximum available anaerobic power level for periods exceeding short power peaks, the

anaerobic lactic acid system is turned on fully. But even beyond this point, the aerobic power output may continue to increase. The usual way of representing the phenomenon of simultaneous aerobic and anaerobic power development is by means of the illustration Fig. 8.2.

Especially if you want to develop your sprinting and climbing powers, as well as an increased resistance to pain, you will at times want to exceed the anaerobic threshold — i.e. the level where anaerobic power becomes a significant factor in power generation. One of the most effective ways to develop the capacity of your power plant is by pushing this level up higher as the result of frequently exceeding it. In addition, anaerobic capacity and muscle strength can be increased by exercising at such high output levels.

Power Versus Speed

Finally in this chapter, let us consider the output levels that are possible and the speeds that may be attained in bicycling for speed. This is done by comparing the available power with the findings from Chapter 7. First, consider the sprinter who delivers 1000 watt, to ride the 200m in a little more than 10 seconds: he'll reach a speed of 70km/h (45 mph).

For longer duration work, you may compare the graphs from the previous chapter with the performance figures for various output levels given in this chapter. This will give you an idea of the speeds and accelerations that may be reached under various conditions by cyclists of different strength levels.

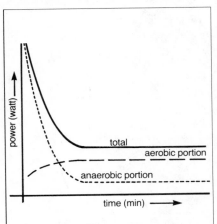

Fig. 8.2 Proportions of aerobic and anaerobic power as a function of time and output level

9. Your Muscles at Work

There is a lot more to cycling than cardiovascular fitness alone. As important as the body's overall capacity to do work at adequate intensity, is the ability of individual muscles to deliver power to the bicycle's drivetrain. In this chapter, we shall take a close look at the muscles involved and at the way any muscle operates. Understanding the way the muscles work, knowing which muscles are involved in cycling and what will increase the muscle's strength, allows the cyclist to gear his training program to maximize muscle power and efficiency.

The illustration Fig. 9.1 shows the human body's muscles from a bicycling perspective. Identified are all those muscles that play a part while pedaling the bicycle, including those that are merely stressed while cycling, without necessarily being in motion. As will be apparent from the illustration, you don't cycle with your leg muscles alone.

Muscles constitute more than one third of an average trained cyclist's body weight; untrained individuals tend to have less muscle weight relative to their total weight. Like other parts of the body, so the muscles too consist of cells, which in this case contain about 70% water. About half the dry muscle weight consists of protein, the rest is made up

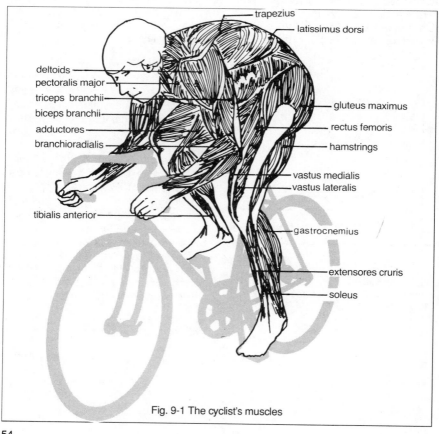

Fig. 9-1 The cyclist's muscles

of approximately equal parts of fats and carbohydrates.

There are two basic types of muscles: the rather flat and smooth autonomously operating ones, which contain the body's various organs, and the more cylindrically shaped voluntary muscles with a striped surface, which respond to the human will. The latter are referred to as skeletal muscles, since they attach to bones of the skeleton at both ends and affect movement of these bones relative to one another. The heart can perhaps best be considered as an intermediate form, being of the striped type but operating involuntarily, i.e. not responding to the human will. Only the striped skeletal muscles are of interest in the present discussion.

The skeletal muscles terminate at both ends in one or more flexible but non-elastic tendons, which in turn connect to protrusions on the bones. There is at least one pair of muscles around every one of the skeleton's joints: a flexor on the inside and a stretcher on the outside of the joint, as shown in Fig. 9.2. We'll first take a close look at the way muscles produce work, followed by an analysis of the operation of the muscles most important to cycling,

namely those that allow you to push the cranks around and around.

The Way Muscles Work
Looking close up (Fig. 9.3), each skeletal muscle consists of densely packed bundles of long fibers with a diameter of about 0.1mm (0.004 in) each. These bundles are surrounded by a flexible mantle, called sarcomere, to which the tendons are attached. There are two distinct types of muscle fibers in each bundle: white ones and red ones. The red ones have that color due to the presence of a high proportion of myoglobin, an oxygen storage protein, making them the main carriers of aerobic power.

These red fibers are referred to as slow twitch (ST) fibers, since they take rather long to react to activation impulses (about 100msec). The white fibers have much less myoglobin, and are thus less suitable for aerobic work. They are known as fast twitch (FT) fibers because they react to activation impulses within 20—30msec. The latter are primarily the carriers of anaerobic power.

The proportions of the two types are probably genetically determined, although each can be developed through

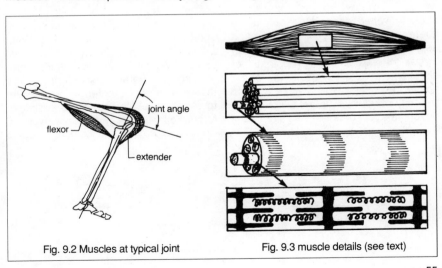

Fig. 9.2 Muscles at typical joint   Fig. 9.3 muscle details (see text)

specific training. A muscle biopsy, removing and analyzing perhaps 20—40mg of muscle fiber from a typical skeletal muscle, can show what the proportions in your muscles are. For do-it-yourselvers, it may be enough to know that long, smooth and relatively slender muscles are those with a predominance of red slow twitch fibers. These are typical for people with good aerobic endurance but limited sprinting capacity. Sprinters tend to have the short and stubbily protruding muscles in which the white fast twitch fibers predominate, giving great anaerobic strength. Typical proportions of red to white (or ST to FT) fibers range from 25/75 for track sprinters to 75/25 for long distance time trialists, 40/60 being about average for non-racers.

Just the same, each type of fiber is capable of some aerobic and some anaerobic work. Specific training probably does not develop only one type of fiber, since the proportions stay the same. And at least one sub-type of the white fast twitch fibers does not appear to respond to any training at all. A training program with a preponderance of short high-power impulses for particular muscles — both on and off the bike — will tend to develop the (anaerobic) strength within either type of muscle fibers. Emphasizing long duration aerobic work in training will tend to increase the aerobic strength potential of either type of fibers. Thus, it may for example be possible to increase aerobic capacity of your white fast twitch fibers beyond that of someone else's red slow twitch fibers.

What we have looked at as a single muscle fiber so far is in reality a complex structure, itself consisting of millions of minute fibers, called myofibrils. These are the actual carriers of muscle work. Each myofibril consists of bundles of long, parallel, mutually overlapping complex protein cells of two different types, called actin and myosin, respectively (see Fig. 9.4). Wherever the two types of fibers overlap, we recognize the darker areas of the striped pattern so characteristic of skeletal muscles.

In the relaxed muscle state, the actin cells protrude relatively far beyond the ends of the matching myosin cells. Projections on the myosin cells act as little hooks that allow the two types of cells to interact. That happens when an electric impulse is sent through the nerve, which in turn releases enzymes to move the projection on the myosin towards the actin cell. As the protrusion moves over, ATP is disintegrated, releasing energy to move the protrusion back to its original position. Upon receiving an impulse, a number of protrusions tense up, pulling the actin cells further in towards the center of the corresponding myosin cell.

This movement can only take place in one direction, namely the direction that shortens or contracts the muscle. With this action, each of the myofibrils tends to be shortened from both ends, contracting the overall muscle length. The muscle will only shorten if the muscle force exceeds the external resisting force. You will note that muscle work is

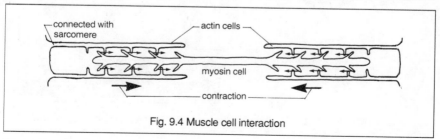

Fig. 9.4 Muscle cell interaction

done whenever the cell protrusions are tensing up, even if the external resistance is so great that the muscle cannot shorten.

If the muscle is shortened we speak of concentric work, if it stays equally long of isometric work, and if it is actually lengthened by the extraneous force of eccentric work. Muscle work is done in each case, even though the mechanical effect is only positive in the case of concentric work, while it is zero for isometric, and negative in the case of eccentric work.

If a stronger muscle force is required, the nerve impulses must be strong, activating many of the myofibril mechanisms, and the muscle must be capable of quickly breaking up ATP. Each action is only brief, at the end of which each myofibril would relax with its actin and myosin cells in their original relative positions, resulting in an untensioned muscle. To achieve continuous muscle tension, a prolonged sequence of impulses must be given. Each myofibril action applies pressure to the blood vessels within the muscles. This results in a surge of blood upon relaxation, allowing the blood to quickly bring fresh stores of oxygen and fuel to the muscle.

Keep in mind that aerobic work is done primarily by the red slow twitch fibers and their energy source is the ATP formed in the mitochondria during the oxygen process. The food for the an aerobic work performed mainly by the white fast twitch fibers is exclusively the ATP formed via the lactic acid system.

Doing lots of work to increase your aerobic muscle strength is not going to have much effect on your sprinting power. This ability depends primarily on your anaerobic power and the proportion and strength of the fast twitch muscle fibers. Conversely, even if you spend all your time doing weight training, resulting in enormously bulky sprinter's muscles, you may not have improved your endurance power, since that depends largely on the aerobic ability and the proportion and strength of your slow-twitch muscle fibers.

Muscle Strength

Though the composition of an individual's muscles, i.e. the ratio of red and white fibers, is largely genetically determined, usage will tend to develop both the muscle's total size and its strength, by increasing the number of fibers. Whereas the ratio cannot be changed, either type of fibers may be developed to work more effectively. In general, muscle training to increase muscle size must involve concentric work, most effectively when at a level close to the maximum muscle force possible, and each training contraction being continued over the maximum range of movement.

It has become increasingly clear in

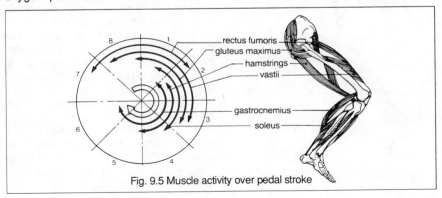

Fig. 9.5 Muscle activity over pedal stroke

recent years that a more specific type of muscle training, involving not the increase of muscle size, but rather of the muscle's efficiency, takes place when the typical movements of the sport are carried out frequently, again preferably close to maximum force level, but (in the case of cycling) at a high speed. The first type of training, which increases bulk and may increase short run strength, appears to lend itself well to weight training methods, while the latter form can only be achieved in actual cycling, even if it takes place on a wind load simulator.

This works well for aerobic muscle strength. It is more difficult to develop anaerobic strength specifically for cycling, though obviously it too can be trained. This capacity is developed by frequently calling on just the kind of work that involves anaerobic output. It is a general observation that many strong anaerobic performers are lazy when it comes to training and do not seem to suffer for it: those blessed with great anaerobic muscle strength will probably get enough benefit from a few hard sprints, while riders who are less well endowed with fast twitch fibers may never get much better at sprinting, however much they work on it.

It has been found that muscles work most effectively when they operate cyclically with short contractions and relatively long relaxation periods. They also deliver more power when they are as it were pre-stressed. Both these points are considerations to keep in mind when determining the appropriate riding style. In cycling, the former condition is satisfied when the legs go through such a motion that different muscle groups take turns in sequence, whereas the second condition is usefully applied when maximum force is required during sprinting, climbing or accelerating, when the legs are restrained by getting out of the saddle or pulling on the arms.

Equally important for muscle effectiveness is their supply of fuel and impulse carrying enzymes. So is the fact that lactic acid and other by-products must be carried off and that small fissures, resulting from excessive use, should not be allowed to inhibit the muscle's operation. For these reasons such factors as the muscle temperature, the enzyme household and the blood circulation must be attuned to the work at hand. Some of these factors are influenced by the food you eat, by warming up before exercise and by massage after strenuous work. In addition, your state of mind and your general state of health probably influence how effective your muscles are at a particular time.

The Cycling Muscles

There are essentially six muscle groups that carry out most of the work involved in propelling the bicycle, as illustrated in Fig. 9.5. It is possible to analyze the nerve impulses in an EMG (electromyograph), to establish which muscle is active at any point in the pedaling cycle. The illustration shows which muscles were thus found to be active during particular sections of the pedaling cycle, which has for convenience been broken down into 8 octants. However, it has not been possible to determine just how much work any particular muscle is performing at any one time.

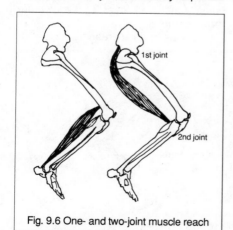

Fig. 9.6 One- and two-joint muscle reach

Let us now take a look at the muscles around just one joint (refer back to Fig. 9.2). As we have seen in the preceding section, the only kind of work a muscle can perform is associated with the tendency to tension and become shorter. Clearly, in each kind of movement only one of the pair of muscles at the joint tightens up, while the other one must be relaxed, or at least it will be forced to become longer. It is of course possible — and wasteful of energy — to tighten both muscles simultaneously, the one restraining the other, as exemplified by the body builder's pose.

When contracted, the flexor tends to bend the joint, the stretcher to straighten it. Though many muscles attach directly to the two neighboring bones of a single joint, some reach beyond the next joint, such as for example the hamstrings at the back of the thigh. Fig. 9.6 shows the two cases simplified for some hypothetical joints, though our present discussion refers to a single joint situation. In fact, the illustrated example, bending the knee, is by no means one of the most demanding tasks in cycling and was selected only because it illustrates the principles involved most clearly.

In reality, it is all even more complex, since not one, but a whole series of different muscles operate during the pedaling cycle, some simultaneously, some overlapping, some at different times. This, in a nutshell, is the reason why so much research has been done to find the optimal position and the optimal pedaling rate. It is also the reason why so much controversy still exists, because it is obviously a very individual matter, which is impossible to capture in a simple rule of thumb that would be valid for all cyclists.

The complexity of the seemingly simple cycling movement can perhaps be appreciated by referring to Fig. 9.5 and observing during which section of the pedal stroke the gastrocnemius is active. This muscle is actually the knee

bender, or flexor, and we've seen that most work is done while extending the knee. When analyzing the movement of the leg in detail, it becomes apparent that during the third octant this muscle must be tensioned to offset other muscle forces that would tend to apply a forward force on the pedal during this part of the stroke.

It will not be necessary to know all the details of muscle movements. But if you are aware that all these things matter, you will be in a good position to know what kind of factors to influence when you find your performance is less than optimal. Experiment carefully and consciously with your posture, your riding style, your pedaling rate and your gearing. Vary the amount of pre-ride warming up, the kind of clothing you wear, the food you eat; try rest, massage, calisthenics and stretching exercises. Experiment around until you have established how to get the most out of your muscles.

Increasing Muscle Strength

Muscles can be strengthened, and they can be made to work more effectively. That is one (but not the only) aspect of training. We've seen before that muscles will tend to grow and become stronger if they are frequently used concentrically at a level close enough to their maximum for longer periods, especially if they are forced to contract over as great a distance as possible. This implies that all muscle training must be dynamic and that no amount of isometric work, by which the muscles are merely held tensely, such as done in stretching exercises, will increase their strength. Muscle training, whether on or off the bike, should involve powerful muscle contractions.

Certain muscles are normally loaded isometrically in cycling, including those of the arms, shoulders and back. So these will not get strengthened by any amount of cycling, even though they can contribute significantly to your cycling strength — at least they will limit your pedaling force if they are not strong enough. To improve these muscles may require weight exercises, loading these particular muscles concentrically over an extended movement, either alone or in combination with other muscles.

That is really the only intelligent use for weight training in preparation for bicycling. Muscle work done in various cycling disciplines is very specific. Speed, duration and sequence of muscle operation, as well as the kind of nerve commands associated with these movements, are unique to cycling. In addition, these motions are really combinations of several overlapping and simultaneous muscle activities, involving a sequence of commands and responses that is impossible to duplicate any other way.

There are even significant differences between cycling at high and at low pedaling speeds, on the level and climbing. Consequently, it is unlikely that weight training and other forms of non-bicycle training will develop the various characteristics (amongst which absolute muscle strength is only one of many) needed for fast, efficient and powerful cycling. This statement may disappoint those who have visions of scientific training as involving lots of machines, instruments and other gadgets.

The scientific approach is not reflected in the equipment you use, but in the conscious observation that helps determine which is the most effective way of training. So far, no better machine has been developed for bicycle training than the one you already have: your bicycle.

10. Food for Cycling and Fitness

There is hardly a subject about which more nonsense has been written and about which more people hold preconceived notions than that of food and diet. So, at the risk of being accused of adding more of the same, here's a whole chapter devoted to the subject of food and drink for cyclists. For an even more thorough (and medically sanctioned) treatment of this material, you are referred to the excellent book *Bicycling Fuel* by Richard Rafoth MD, also published by Bicycle Books.

In cycling circles you will encounter staunch vegetarians and veritable carnivores, carrot munchers and pill poppers, all claiming the key to success lies in the way they fill their belly. Though the subject is not without interest, I would suggest considering it more soberly: forget about fad diets and concentrate on selecting your food consciously.

In America, fitness cyclists seem to largely come from the same ranks as health food freaks and other diet conscious people. Nothing wrong with that, but many of the theories propounded in those circles are only relevant for people with a sedentary lifestyle. However, it makes a great difference whether you spend your day lounging about in an office, a car and at home (even if you do a little fitness cycling three times a week), or spend several hours each day burning up calories on a bicycle. What you need is not a diet but a clear understanding of the function of food as it applies to your performance and overall health. Most of all, you must realize the following facts:

- Although minimal fitness cycling makes no special nutritional demands, long distance cycling requires more calories.
- As for the supposedly superior nutrients, such as proteins and vitamins, even an active athlete does not require more than an inactive person of the same weight.
- More is not necessarily better: If X grams of protein or Y milligrams of some vitamin or mineral are required, then it does not follow that twice these quantities will improve your performance even one bit.

The Tasks of Food

Your body, including every organ, muscle and bone, needs food to function properly. The tasks that must be fulfilled by the things you eat and drink boil down to providing the following:

- Energy to keep the body's temperature at the necessary level for the various systems to operate;
- Energy needed to perform mechanical work by means of muscle action;
- Liquids to conduct heat, control body temperature and sustain various physiological processes;
- Building materials needed to grow and replace cell structures;
- Enzymes that allow the other processes to operate efficiently.

The most important substances to ingest that are necessary or useful to carry out these functions are listed as follows:

- Water
- Carbohydrates
- Fats
- Proteins
- Vitamins
- Mineral trace elements
- Fibers

The following sections will describe each of these major substances, followed by an analysis of the way these food substances fit into the complex of functions that must be fulfilled for the human body to operate effectively, especially under such physically demanding conditions as presented by bicycle training and participation. Finally, some special cases concerning nutrition that are often discussed in cycling circles will be presented.

Water
About 70% of your body weight is water, which serves several different functions. It is the major carrier for other substances in the body and is essential for the process of temperature control. Water must be replenished as it evaporates or is excreted. It needn't always be taken in the form of plain water, since it is contained in most foods, especially in fruits, vegetables and meat. And of course almost any beverage will provide it quickly.

Within the body many substances, such as sugars and minerals, are passed from the water into the cells by means of osmosis. That is the process of filtering through a thin membrane, whereby the transfer is always from the side with the higher concentration to the side with the lower concentration. Consequently, the concentrations of essential substances (e.g. sugar and in some cases table salt) in the water you drink should be just a little higher in the liquid than it is in the body cells. Thus, the way to introduce sugars into the body is to bind them in what is referred to as an isotonic solution, meaning it has at least the same concentration of dissolved materials as the liquid in the body cells. For sugar that means about 2.5%.

Carbohydrates
This predominant energy source, comprising both sugars and starch, is present in virtually all foodstuffs. The difference between sugar and starch is that the latter takes about two hours longer to provide energy, as it must be turned into usable sugar in the digestive system first, while most sugars (especially dextrose) can be taken up in the blood stream very shortly after they are consumed. However nice it may seem

to get something that works quickly, starch-rich foods are to be preferred over sugars, since their effect is not depleted as fast. Besides foods containing starches also provide other essential substances and help keep the body's digestive system in better trim. They should be the staple of the active cyclist's diet.

Particularly rich sources of starch are all grain products and potatoes. Yet starches are also contained in virtually all other vegetable foods and in meat. Natural sugars are contained in most fruits and honey, while refined sugars are provided only too generously by just about all ready-made foods and drinks. Whether natural or refined, all sugars provide energy equally efficiently (ordinary refined sugar at the lowest cost). Though you may want to take a sugared drink for quick energy on the road, try to avoid sugars in your everyday diet, except in the form of fruits and natural juices, which also contain other valuable nutrients and digestive aids.

Fats
Although appropriately derided as a no-good in the inactive person's diet, fats are the most energy-efficient nutrient. However, fats as consumed are slowly digested and converted. Fat is used in the body as a store of energy and an insulator. It's present in meats and dairy products, but also in many nuts and various vegetable sources. The distinction between polysaturated and unsaturated fats is probably not as significant to the endurance cyclist as it is to the less active.

It is probably true that the majority of people in the western world have accumulated too much fat. But it is very hard to avoid eating it altogether, since it is tied up with proteins in so many products that we have grown fond of. The tender American steak contains twice as much fat as the tougher stuff consumed in the rest of the world, and it will be hard to convince most people they don't need to eat as much meat as they do, or that less tender meat would be better for them.

In the body, fat is used as an energy source in the form of free fatty acids (FFA). These are carried in the blood stream and are used much like sugar for energy. As consumed, the fat first builds up as padding in various places, to be released in the form of FFA as needed to supply energy when work must be done at a certain level. This will be covered in more detail under *Food for Energy* below.

Proteins
Proteins are the building blocks for cell growth and maintenance. They comprise various combinations of a group of aminoacids contained in many foods, but especially in meats, fish and dairy products, as well as — though in lesser concentrations — in legumes and grains. For the body to use proteins for cell building, the aminoacids must be present during any one meal in a certain ratio, which is most closely approximated by egg white, fish and meat. Other forms of protein foods are only adequately efficient if eaten in some combination of various types, e.g. legumes with potatoes, bread with milk, or beans with rice.

Contrary to popular belief, athletes don't need more protein than other people of the same age and body weight. For each kg body weight only about 1g of protein is required per day. Slightly more may be needed by growing youngsters and during the initial building-up phase of training, when the muscles are developing. Most American adults get at least three times as much protein as they need.

Excess proteins, i.e. those not used for cell building, are simply burned up to provide energy, much like carbohydrates. A crying shame, since proteins are on average 5 times as expensive and considerably harder to digest. For the latter reason, protein-rich meals should not be eaten during or shortly before demanding organized events or training rides. Breakfast and lunch should be heavy on starches and low on fats and protein, while the best time to eat meals containing more protein is perhaps about 6—7 PM: Late enough not to interfere with demanding physical activity, yet early enough to be largely digested before the night.

Vitamins
Primarily a number of acids that are required in small amounts to provide the enzymes necessary for operation of various functions. Vitamins are distinguished into water soluble and fat soluble ones. The water-soluble vitamins (B and C) leave the body fast, so they must be taken in daily, while the fat-soluble ones (A, D, E and K) can be stored in the body over longer periods. Various vitamins are contained mainly in fresh fruits and vegetables, organ meats

Table 10-1 Comparison of carbohydrates, fats and protein as energy sources

food type	energy content		respiration quotient	typical time to digest
	(kJ/g)	(kcal/g)	RQ (CO_2/O_2)	(hours)
carbohydrate	17.2	4.1	1.0	
sugars				0.1–2
starch				2–3
fat	38.9	9.3	0.7	6–8
protein	17.2	4.1		6–8

and whole grain products. A well balanced and varied diet will provide all the essential vitamins you ever need.

Consequently, there is probably no need for vitamin supplements if you include these foods in your diet, and there is no need to take vitamin tablets during even the hardest rides. Especially the fat-soluble vitamins should be taken in moderation to avoid large build-ups with questionable effects on your health. The water-soluble vitamins B and C, being necessary for energy production in the body, may have to be supplemented if performance falls off and no other cause is evident. Since any excess of these is excreted, there is no risk of getting too much. In rare cases you may benefit by taking modest doses of multi- vitamin tablets on a regular basis, for example if you are for some reason not able to adhere to a well balanced food intake.

Minerals

Also referred to as electrolytes, some minerals are required in small quantities for enzyme functions. Those only required in the minutest amounts are referred to as trace elements. Most are present mainly in vegetables, some fruits and grains. The most familiar of these elements is the sodium which becomes free when ordinary table salt dissolves in water. Others, such as potassium, calcium, and iron (the latter needed as a carrier of oxygen in blood and slow twitch muscle fiber cells) are equally needed.

Since these electrolytes are water-soluble, their excess is excreted with urine and perspiration. Consequently, after a very long and hard ride in hot weather, a case may be made for their replacement if heavy perspiration has depleted their level below the minimum required concentration in the body.

Back in the early seventies a smart businessman decided to analyze perspiration and offer a drink containing all the elements lost that way. No medical evidence has ever been presented to support the need for this, but that has not stopped dozens of manufacturers from introducing expensive and awful tasting liquids containing too much sugar and useless electrolytes. Nor has it discouraged millions of cyclists from buying and — what is worse — drinking this junk.

Most electrolyte drinks are totally unnecessary, of course: the water and sugar can be provided in a more appetizing form and better balanced proportions, while the only electrolytes that matter can be replenished by adding some table salt and eating a banana. Beyond that, a reasonably balanced diet will take care of all your electrolyte needs and is the healthiest way to eat.

Table 10-2 Comparison of typical digestion times for various foods

time in stomach	food types
1–2 hours	water, coffee, tea, boiled rice, soft boiled egg, fresh water fish
2–3 hours	milk, coffee with cream, boiled or baked potatoes, low-fiber cooked vegetables, fruit, white bread, hard boiled egg, omelette or fried egg, salt water fish, veal
3–4 hours	whole grain bread, fried or French fried potatoes, fried rice, fibrous vegetables (e.g. spinach), salads (without dressing), beef, ham, boiled tender chicken
4–5 hours	beans, high-fiber vegetables, boiled or fried meat, poultry and game
6–8 hours	mushrooms, bacon, sardines in oil

Fibers

Fibrous materials, which are contained largely in unprocessed vegetable and grain products, are necessary to stimulate the operation of the digestive system. With the exercise of your training program, you will not need it as much as most sedentary folks, but you may not get enough to feel well. Cycling with clogged intestines is not very efficient and enjoyable. Again, the famous balanced diet, with whole grain bread instead of the white pulp usually dished up in most households, cooked and raw vegetables and various fruits will keep you well supplied. If not, use bran cereals or add bran flakes to other foods.

Food for Energy

The overwhelming majority of the food you eat will be used to provide energy — both the heat energy to keep your body warm and the mechanical energy that allows you to do muscle work. Carbohydrates, fat and proteins all lend themselves to that purpose. They can all be converted into the glucose that is transported in the blood or the glycogen that may be stored in the liver and muscle tissue. Thus, they can ultimately all be burned to form the ATP that constitutes the raw material for muscle work. However, these three foods are not all equally efficient, and they require different proportions of oxygen to perform their task. Furthermore, different kinds of foods — even with similar constituents — require longer or shorter digestion periods before they can be used effectively. Table 10–1 summarizes the major differences between the three basic energy sources, while Table 10–2 may help you get some feel for the time it takes the body to digest certain foodstuffs.

The amount of work expended and the food energy consumed can best be measured in kJ, which stands for kilo-Joules. To relate this to more familiar units, 4.2kJ = 1kcal, which is what's really meant when Calories are referred to in older works about nutrition. An average person leading a quiet life needs about 7000kJ of energy a day. A hard day's cycling will add anything up to 4500kJ of mechanical energy.

Considering the human engine's efficiency of approx. 0.25, that means an additional 18000kJ must be provided, adding up to a total daily energy requirement of about 24000kJ. That is also just about the maximum your body can take up in a day. Any energy expended in excess of this (that happens in heavy mountain stages of the Tour de France and similar races) will go at the expense of your body weight. Yet eating more than enough to supply that food will not even make you fatter: it goes straight through your system.

On the other hand, if you follow a minimal — or even a moderate — fitness regimen, don't expect to get anywhere close to these levels of energy consumption. Half an hour's or even a whole hour's cycling at a good pace still is nothing like racing all day. So you may have to be more concerned about eating too much than bout getting enough food to last.

As you can tell from table 10–1, fats are easily the most energy efficient nutrient, offering twice as much energy per gram as either carbohydrates or protein. The fat you burn passes into the system as free fatty acids (FFA). That's not the fat you have just eaten, but derives from the stuff that has accumulated in various places on the body. These fat stores are formed by all excess foods not needed for immediate energy supply, which is always converted into fat, except if it exceeds the maximum digestive limit mentioned above. At most levels of output the body uses a combination of free fatty acids and glycogen for aerobic energy production: mainly fat at low levels, mainly glycogen at higher levels, as represented in Fig. 10.1. Note that the range is rather wide, individuals differing somewhat. The typical female body tends to favor fat metabolism; for any athlete, a shift towards fat metabolism occurs as an effect of aerobic training.

It is possible to determine which proportions of the energy comes from fat and carbohydrate metabolisms, respectively, at any time. This is done by comparing the volumes of exhaled carbon dioxide and inhaled oxygen, called the respiratory quotient RQ. If RQ is 1:1 all energy comes from carbohydrates, if it is all comes from 0.7 from fat. Any intermediate ratio allows the physiologist to determine in what ratio fat and carbohydrates are being burned. On really long exhausting rides, such as mountainous stage races and double centuries, the supply of carbohydrates is in danger two ways. At high output levels it is used up first and fastest, and its supply is limited to what can be taken up by the body in a day. You may run out before the end of the ride.

No such problems at low output levels, such as touring and moderate fitness cycling, where free fatty acids are preferably burned. The supply of fat on even the leanest body will probably suffice to cycle half way around the world at a modest speed. But for the road racer, who has to keep up a murderous pace all day and still have enough power left for a dash or a climb, the supply problem may become evident. Anywhere beyond 75% of $\dot{V}_{O2max}$ he'll be burning virtually only carbohydrates, as evidenced by an RQ close to 1.0. The glycogen in liver and muscles, the glucose in the blood and the food in the belly are the only energy supplies available, and once these are gone, it's all over.

The obvious way to prolong the energy supply is by reducing the pace to a level below 75% $\dot{V}_{O2max}$ as much of the time as possible. That's one good reason to take it easier by riding in an echelon. This reduces the wind resistance enough to make all the difference on a long fast ride. Another technique to maximize the fat burning, as evidenced by a low RQ, is simply to do more training at continuously high output levels. This tends to shift the balance more towards the fat metabolism. Finally, some researchers (and many cyclists) feel the fat metabolism can be stimulated by taking caffeine.

Everything in moderation though: probably not more than 4mg per kg of body weight (2mg per lb). That is the equivalent of about two small cups of strong coffee at the beginning of a ride

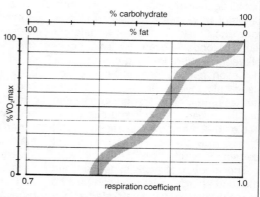

The respiratory quotient RQ is used as an indicator to establish to what extent energy is generated by burning carbohydrates and fat respectively. Up to about 75% of $\dot{V}_{O2max}$, the low value for RQ indicates that most energy is provided by fat metabolism. To maximize endurance, economize on available food, and to encourage weight reduction, try to stay within that range as much as possible.

Fig. 10.1 Respiration Quotient (RQ): fat versus carbohydrate use during exercise

for the average body. Anybody who drinks more at any time or who takes strong caffeinated drinks just before the end of a ride is fooling himself, since it can have no positive effect. Even when used as suggested here there is a problem with caffeine, since it works as a diuretic, i.e. it encourages liquids to leave the body in the form of urine. Consequently, in hot weather, particularly for rides involving a lot of climbing, the use of caffeine may be dangerous: you will need all the water you can drink to act as a cooling medium.

Carbohydrate Loading

That's a technique used by some athletes who have to perform well in 2 hour duration activity only once in a blue moon. It's no use for short or really long rides, nor for stage races, and dubious at best even for its intended purpose. The idea, is to exercise to exhaustion several days well before the big events, after which you start eating carbohydrates in generous supplies, without doing very much in the way of hard work. The assumption is that the muscles will absorb lots of carbohydrates in the form of energy carrying glycogen.

For bicycling it is a highly questionable technique, especially if one considers that muscle glycogen stores never satisfy the bulk of your long duration energy requirements anyway. If it works at all, then only for competitive events over time periods of about 2 hours — neither much longer, nor much shorter. In addition, chances are that the benefit of continued training in the days leading up to the event would have been greater to your performance, as they certainly are to your overall long term condition. You can try it, but you may find the results to be negative.

The Role of Water

Water is quite essential to the body's proper operation. This contrary to at least one European cycling myth which claims that drier is faster. That statement may apply to the English time trialists who ride 25 miles in 50—60 minutes on a cold day, after which they may indulge in all the beer they can down before the pubs close. But it is nonsense when we are considering any intensive activity of several hours duration, especially in hot weather.

Water is tied up in the body with several other substances, for which it acts as a carrier. It is particularly important for regulating the body's temperature. During vigorous cycling in hot weather the cyclist may lose water faster than he can possibly drink it. Half a liter, or about one pint, an hour is all the body will absorb, while it may evaporate at twice that rate. To keep the body at the optimal temperature for muscular and mental work, water is used. Whenever the temperature threatens to get too high, the pores and sweat glands are opened and sweat is excreted, the natural evaporation of which will cool the body.

Especially in warm weather and on long exhausting rides, you will therefore need more water than you can carry in bottles on the bike. Start drinking well before the start, and drink frequently in moderate quantities during the ride. Allow perspiration to evaporate, rather than wiping it off. Since water is also an excellent medium to tie up sugars and electrolytes isotonically, it is frequently suggested to carry two bottles on a hot and exhausting ride: one with plain water for cooling, the other with a water based mixture containing at least 2.5% sugar and up to a teaspoonful of table salt per pint. Personally, I prefer natural fruit juice over this man-made mix. It serves the same purpose but tastes a lot better.

Weight Reduction

The quickest, easiest, healthiest and cheapest way to improve your performance may well be by reducing your weight. That's assuming you are like most people, who carry unnecessary ballast in the form of excess fat. Good endurance cyclists are lean. They have body fat percentages not exceeding 8% and 12% respectively for men and women. The higher optimal fat percentage for women corresponds nicely with the previously observed phenomenon of their more active fat metabolism.

The body fat percentage can be determined by means of several techniques, most simply by measuring certain skin folds, which any sports physician or paramedic can do. If you are determined to lose weight, don't try to force it in a period of high physical demands, and don't try to do it only by eating less. Use a combination of various techniques. Eat less and differently, taking more fibrous matter and less fats and sugars; do more physical work in addition to your training — use your bike instead of the car, the stairs instead of the elevator.

A Cyclist's Meal Planner
It is possible to eat adequately without any other advice than that contained in the preceding paragraphs, and perform admirably, even in competitive cycling. However, for those who prefer some additional guidance, here are some specific hints on how one might divide the required food intake over a cycling day. All this assuming you cycle a lot, not just the minimum of 20 minutes a day needed to maintain cardiovascular fitness, but regular long distance rides. If you ride just a little, you should eat the same but much less of it.

Breakfast:
Aim for a high starch intake, combined with vitamins, fibers and minerals and modest amounts of proteins, avoiding sugars and fat. Fruit or fruit juice; whole grain cereal with e.g. banana or dried fruit and low fat milk or natural plain yoghurt, whole grain bread. Try to eat breakfast at least an hour before a demanding event or training ride.

Lunch:
If your day is an active one, including a long, hard ride in the afternoon, aim for a relatively light lunch after a big breakfast, again containing more starch than proteins and avoiding fats and sugars. Eat salad with bread or other starch foods, combined with small quantities of e.g. meat or cheese. A sandwich should not be lots of meat or cheese with a little bread, but rather lots of bread with little meat or cheese — 'breadwiches' is what my cycling companions disparagingly call the food that keeps me going while they stuff themselves with fat and proteins. Drink low fat milk and have a dessert of plain yoghurt or fruit.

Supper:
This is rightly your heaviest meal and the one time to include more protein foods, though it will still be preferable to go easy on tender (read: high-fat) meats. In addition to meat or other protein foods, eat generous quantities of starches and fresh or cooked vegetables and fruit. Drink natural fruit juice or low fat milk. Hold off on salad dressings, gravies and sauces. Try to have dinner relatively early in the evening. Get some light exercise, even if it is only a 20 minute walk, after dinner to help digestion.

Snacks:
If the urge strikes during the day, the active athlete can indulge in snacks between meals. In fact, it will be even wiser to eat six small meals than three big ones, if one does a lot of hard riding. When eating between meals, avoid junk food, though. Instead of sugared and fatty stuff, choose any of the relatively light foods that give you something to munch on, contain starch, fibers, minerals and vitamins. Eat fresh or dried fruit, crackers, raw vegetables and yoghurt; drink water, tea, low fat milk or natural fruit juice.

11. Improving Your Endurance

Cycling in all its most popular forms is an endurance sport *par excellence*. One hundred mile rides (called centuries in club cycling circles) and even multiples of that distance (referred to as double and triple centuries) are so common that the cycling publications can't list all of them each weekend during the season.

What would be considered a monumental achievement in any other sport is taken for granted in cycling. At the competitive level cycling is about twice as fast as running. So, since the 26 mile marathon is the toughest and longest event in running, one might expect the toughest bike races to be perhaps 50—60 miles, and a typical race rather more like 10 miles. Not so: since over a century much longer distances and durations have dominated competitive cycling, even though short track events have their followers too.

The bicycle lends itself superbly to duration work. Whereas the runner must remain active all the time to continue moving at all, the momentum gained in cycling allows occasional coasting, and riding with significantly reduced power output does not immediately result in an equally obvious drop in speed. Since cycling motions are gradual without severe impact or strain, if done correctly, even the longest races need not cause the kind of damage to muscles, joints and tendons that wipes out marathon runners for up to a week after competition.

Long duration events are of course overwhelmingly aerobic. At a low enough level, aerobic activity could be continued almost perpetually, allowing for little more than interruptions for feeding, sleep and some of nature's other demands. That is simply because at such a low level nothing very much more demanding takes place than keeping heart and lungs going to supply the muscles with oxygen and nutrients, while the skeletal muscles themselves are never strained to the point of serious exertion.

Even so, the beginning bicyclist on his first long trip, who probably maintains hardly more than a minimal output level, finds himself stopping for rest brakes at increasingly close intervals. After 30 or 40 miles he may be ready to hang his bike in the willows, if only he could figure out how to get home without it. And this person was not even doing any hard work, whereas in organized events and training you will not only pedal, you will also be expected to put in some real effort. So there must be more to endurance on a bicycle than meets the eye.

Factors in Bicycle Endurance

There are a number of distinct factors that govern endurance while cycling, which shall be covered in the following sections. Throughout your initial training and riding efforts, the emphasis will shift from one factor to the next, as your training progress helps you overcome the restrictions formed by the more elementary ones, and you start reaching the subsequent higher hurdles. Nobody, except some rarely talented and already fit athlete, achieves all this progress in a single season: be prepared to work on it for at least one year of preparation and one or two seasons of participation.

The very first factor that limits bicycling endurance, even at a minimal output level, is simply the motion of cycling. Three distinct characteristics of various types of motions are at work here. The beginning cyclist referred to in the example has probably overcome none of these yet, even if we assume he has mastered an even more elementary skill, namely that of finding the right posture on the bike, as was outlined in Chapter 2.

First there is simply the repeated movement of the legs, which must become virtually autonomous for really competent cycling. Slowly the beginner will have to build up his skill to progress from a conscious 'push, push' via an equally conscious 'round- and-round' to a smooth and automatic form of this same cyclical leg movement. Even so, at first it can only be maintained for a limited period of time: to keep it up for many hours demands having practiced it during even more hours at a stretch. It's a skill that can in part be mastered through many hours of riding a wind load simulator, but must also be trained on the road.

Then there is the complex of actions necessary to keep the bicycle balanced and following its intended course. It involves quick decisions and reactions on the road. Things like that occupy the mind of the beginning cyclist to the point of mental and physical overload. As time progresses and as you experience miles and hours in the saddle, many of the necessary thoughts, actions and reactions will leave pre-programmed paths in your nervous system.

Only when that point is reached will your cycling skills have developed to the level where purely physical factors determine your endurance. To achieve that, there is no substitute for riding the bike on the road under a wide range of conditions, ranging from fast and winding mountain roads to densely trafficked urban streets to precipitous trails. The final touch will be added in your first season of group riding, surrounded by a bunch of others even more incompetent than you and seemingly out to kill one another.

The last stage of motion control is that associated with taking the right actions to adapt to varying conditions. That's not just a matter of physical environment, but includes your own condition. Once you have gained enough cycling experience, you will be able to almost subconsciously react the right way to signals from your own mind and body, as well as the outside factors demanding a change of gear, a change in the pace, the need for a drink or a bite. Sounds silly perhaps, but incompetent cyclists lose much of their endurance potential thinking about such simple actions, which the more experienced competitor makes correctly without either thought or loss of time. This is another skill that can only be developed with the bike on the road, and requires conscious attention until these things actually become automatic.

Endurance at High Output Levels

Even if long distance cycling is largely an aerobic exercise, it is often done at a certain elevated speed, both in organized events and while training. To maintain this higher speed, the rider's aerobic capacity must be greater. One reason why beginning cyclists often fail to maintain a speed for any length of time is their inadequate aerobic capacity, which may be hidden by strong muscles and relatively high anaerobic capacity during shorter exercises. Thus many seemingly promising riders fail to maintain the set pace, even though they are remarkably powerful on shorter distances.

To avoid draining anaerobic energy in the early stages of a longer ride, the aerobic potential must be raised as high as possible. Not only would an early recourse to anaerobic systems soon deplete them, their lactic acid generation and oxygen debt problems would actually inhibit the remaining aerobic potential. The result would be a reduction both in speed and in endurance at any speed. Consequently, the cyclist must try to raise his aerobic power so high that there is minimal need to tap the anaerobic sources. This is achieved by consciously keeping a regular pace, thus avoiding the need for acceleration. In addition, training many miles at an output level close to the aerobic threshold will tend to raise that limit high enough to avoid passing it.

All high intensity work involves a certain amount of anaerobic work as well. This is the APT-CP system, which is activated whenever higher muscle forces are required to provide the short muscle power peaks. No lactic acid is generated, but this system too is distinct from the regular aerobic one that runs on nothing but glucose and oxygen. Like the major anaerobic lactic acid system, it activates the fast-twitch muscle fibers. Training to maintain this work up for extended periods will probably also be a key to endurance work at high power output levels.

It cannot be claimed with absolute certainly, but it is probably possible to increase the effectiveness of this system, if not to actually increase the number of fast-twitch fibers. Requisites are both an optimally functioning enzyme household and frequent practice in using this system. Here are the factors that positively influence the enzyme household controlling the effectiveness of the system:

- a balanced diet with enough essential vitamins and minerals;
- pre-ride warm-up and proper clothing for temperature control;
- sufficient liquid intake before and during the activity;
- a positive mental attitude.

Long Distance Cycling and Pain
Cycling far and fast may hurt. It is part of the macho image of bicycling, but it is also true that some people either do not suffer pain or have achieved, not (as some think) to ignore the pain, but to prevent it through training. Limiting the pain you feel will probably greatly increase your endurance at any higher output.

The pain threshold is the amount of exposure to pain where it is first noticed. It is probably at the same level for all people, man or woman, cyclists or not.

But there are degrees of hurting: putting your hand in boiling water causes more pain than it does in 60 degrees C (140 degrees F), though the pain threshold is exceeded in either case. Somewhere beyond this threshold there must be a pain limit, beyond which one cannot endure pain, however much you grit your teeth.

That upper limit can be changed to a higher or lower level. When you're sick you are more sensitive, whereas either a positive outlook or fear may enable you to endure more. Then there is medication (or drugs, to call a spade a bloody shovel), primarily a group of alkaloids referred to as opiates. As it turns out, the human brain produces a form of proteins known as neuropeptides, that — though different in chemical makeup — are identical in their spatial form and structure. At least one of these, beta-endorphine, has the same pain suppressing effect as e.g. morphine.

People with high levels of beta-endorphine are more resistant to pain. It seems many women have higher levels of this than most men (that makes reference to toughness as being a macho quality rather ironic), and there are significant differences between individuals of the same sex. But even within the same body the level is not constant, increasing with extended exercise, although it falls off again after a couple of hours. Though not definitely proven, it appears that a regular training regimen tends to increase the normal level of beta-endorphine in the blood. Thus, one way to attain greater endurance at a level that would at first hurt, is to train regularly for extended periods of time. This is additional to the direct training effect that increases the available power.

The Bonk as a Limit to Endurance
During extended rides at high output levels many riders experience a point where their body just lets them down.

This experience is referred to as the bonk and feels at least as unsettling as it sounds: muscle and stomach cramps, feelings of heaviness in the legs and emptiness in the stomach, and a general giddy weakness. To endure on a long tough ride, you must avoid reaching this point, or at least to overcome it quickly once it does arrive.

Though popular belief amongst cyclists has it that this phenomenon is simply the result of the depletion of glucose in the blood, it is in fact much more complex. Besides, it is not merely a physical problem, since much of it must be attributed to loss of coordination in the brain and nervous system (this being indeed the result of glucose depletion, since that is the only form of energy the brain can use). Any one, or several, of the following causes may be involved:

- dehydration;
- overheating;
- low blood glucose;
- depletion of muscle glycogen;
- excessive lactic acid level;
- loss of minerals or electrolytes.

All these factors have something to do with nutrition. In addition to following the advice on nutrition in Chapter 10, in particular taking enough liquids, especially in hot weather, your physical and mental fitness also has a great effect. Even the healthy, well trained athlete may at some point experience the bonk, but only after a much longer period of hard riding. Try to train over the same distance as your longest organized ride at least once a week. That training ride must be absolved at a comparable level of exertion to prevent this humiliating experience from striking in an organized ride with others.

Prevention is the only true cure, but there are a few things you can do when it hits you. When you do feel the bonk, don't try to push yourself harder, but choose a lower gear without speeding up the pedaling rate. Your riding speed and muscle force will fall back to a more comfortable level. Once you recover, you may be able to make up for lost time. Take liquid glucose nourishment, containing adequate quantities of sugar and salt: 5—10% sugar and up to a half teaspoonful of table salt per liter (about one quart). Half a bottle of this mixture every 15 minutes or so (or about half that much to prevent the problem in the first place) may do the trick. It won't give you magical endurance or strength, and is better to do before you reach this point, but it will relatively soon bring your nervous system under control, allowing you at least to use what physical strength you still have. Continuing at a modest pace will get you home safely and may even lead to recoverye.

12. Basic Training Theory

Whether for fitness or competition, the ultimate purpose of training is to improve condition and performance. Training theory is the summary of the results of investigations into the various ways this goal may be reached.

Eventually, these theoretical findings must be turned into practical training methods and adapted to what suits the individual cyclist as it fits in with his or her other activities. Chapters 13 and 14 are devoted to the practical training methods for on-the-road and indoor training, respectively. The aspect of planning for individual needs will be covered in Chapter 15. The present chapter, on the other hand, provides the theoretical basis for what follows.

The overall concept of training is not limited to physical exercise alone. Correctly, it should include all methods that lend themselves to the improvement of athletic performance. Though most of the attention in this and the two following chapters is rightly focussed on various exercises, other aspects must be considered too. To give but one example, consider that the most universal measure of aerobic capacity, and in-

directly of duration cycling performance, is $\dot{V}_{O2max}$. As explained in Chapter 13, this measure relates oxygen capacity per unit of time to body weight. Consequently, a change in body weight will affect $\dot{V}_{O2max}$. You may well be able to increase $\dot{V}_{O2max}$ by e.g. 5% if you can reduce your body weight by the same percentage, assuming you were carrying unneeded fat, as probably 90% of all Americans are.

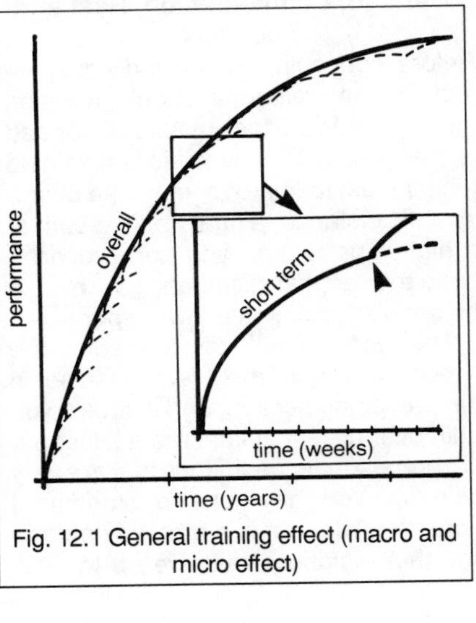

Fundamental to all training theory are the identification of trainability and the various specific training effects. The former will help you identify where and when training will afford the greatest improvement. The latter allows you to establish which methods must be used to develop specific aspects of overall performance. Primarily, the overall training effect will be an improved performance due to exercise. This can be represented graphically as shown in Fig. 12.1: the improvement is quite dramatic at first, then tapers off as you get closer to your limits as they apply to the specific ability exercised and the method used. An important distinction would be between those effects that influence the athlete's overall condition and those that work on specific discipline-related abilities.

Training Effects

Perhaps the most essential factor to improve is the overall condition — certainly during the first period of training for bicycle performance improvement. This can be seen as the ability to perform any kind of work through the output of physiological power. That may be either aerobic or anaerobic or, more typically, a combination of the two that matches the demands of the particular discipline. In long distance cycling, we are talking primarily, though not exclusively, of aerobic power. Anaerobic power is most needed for sprinting, both as a distinct

Fig. 12.1 General training effect (macro and micro effect)

track discipline and as the essential component that allows a rider to get ahead of the pack, catch up with it, get across an intersection before the light turns red, or storm up a steep hill.

Training Specificity

One particularly important condition for effective training — and also one that is frequently ignored by those who are looking for shortcuts — is specificity of training. Simply put, it amounts to training just the kind of thing you will be doing in the course of the type of rides you are preparing for. To be a bicyclist, train on a bicycle. To train for long distances, ride long distances in training; to ride in the mountains, train in the mountains. I realize that actual conditions cannot always be duplicated in training. In that case, use some imagination to come up with good simulations of the conditions sought.

Discipline-specific training effects have more to do with the particular movements peculiar to bicycling. Although most of these are common to all bicycle riding at speed, some can be distinguished according to the kind of riding for which they are important. In the following sections, I shall keep the discussion as general as possible, merely reminding the reader to consider each time which particular effects are the more important ones for his or her personal situation. In this connection it should be pointed out that it is established practice in bicycling to train for all possible types of riding. Though it may be appropriate to emphasize certain skills, you will probably never be successful in cycling by training only for one specialty or the other.

Going from the general to the more specific, a list of desired training effects would include the following:

- increase cardiorespiratory capacity to maximize aerobic output;
- raise the anaerobic threshold;

- increase anaerobic power;
- increase endurance;
- increase efficiency of movement;
- increase power and speed of essential muscles;
- increase power of restraining muscles.

Somewhere in the preceding chapters each of these points has cropped up. Here we shall look at them more specifically, with the purpose of establishing and systematizing the training techniques most suitable for each of these desired effects.

Consider, though, that the total is not necessarily the sum of the parts: it may be more or less. In some cases, increasing one aspect may have an immediate positive effect on total performance. In other cases it does not work out that simply. Developing muscle force, for example, may not have any effect on your cycling performance if that is not the limiting factor, but e.g. your capacity to perform aerobic work. Thus it should be obvious that you must work on all effects simultaneously, always emphasizing the factor that limits your performance most at that time.

Overload, Compensation, Rest and Recovery

Before continuing to the individual effects to be trained, I should mention these very important factors. Overload is the basis of many effective training techniques: to improve your time over a specific distance, aim at training both at a higher pace than you can presently handle over that distance, and over a higher distance, if at a lower speed.

This may seem to contradict the specificity requirement emphasized in the preceding section, and it does if you train over distances that are a lot longer or shorter, under conditions that are very different. You may have to experiment around a little, but it is probably safe to say that distances that are up to 10%

longer and speeds that are up to 5% higher are reasonable.

The compensation effect is the ability of the body's systems to recover from an elevated load by overcompensating to the point that it allows a subsequent higher output level. This same effect is at work in mechanisms ranging from short term interval training to peaking programs during weeks preceding a major event. This is essentially the same principle that makes carbohydrate loading work.

In each of these methods, the body is first depleted in a particularly strenuous regimen, followed by a period of recovery. Before the system reaches its normal condition, a period of increased capacity is reached, and the principle of all these methods is to exploit this period. The principle is shown in Fig. 12.2. The benefit lies in the ability to accept a higher workload during that time, allowing e.g. increased training intensity (in the short run) or a superior competitive performance (in the long run) or the ability to store greater quantities of glucose (in the case of carbohydrate loading).

The recovery period between the last peak and the subsequent increased performance is quite individual and must be established by experiment for each rider. Somewhere a balance must be established, where the overcompensation resulting from the preceding exertion is still significant, while at the same time the body is rested enough to work efficiently.

It has been found that recovery is also necessary between days with very extensive exercise. Avoid training very hard or long on consecutive days, unless it is specifically geared towards depletion in connection with the long-term compensation effect. To achieve optimal performance, the entire training and participation program must be periodized, i.e. scheduled over various time periods: a micro and a macro cycle. This system should also consider the phenomenon shown in the short cycle curves of Fig. 12.1: when the improvement due to training one system reaches the limit, the next period should set in with a different emphasis.

Rest is also a form of recovery, and it plays a role in training and preparation. Actually, a sleepless night is not much less effective in providing physical recovery than deep sleep. The problem is more a psychological one, which may be minimized now that you know that it is not as physiologically devastating to

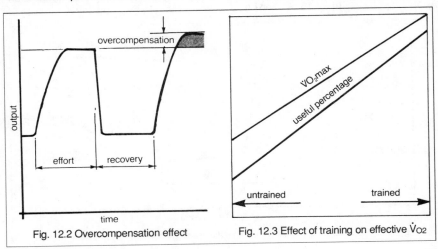

Fig. 12.2 Overcompensation effect   Fig. 12.3 Effect of training on effective $\dot{V}_{O2}$

have a lousy night's sleep. It may also be a consolation to know that it is not the last night, but rather the one preceding it, that has the greatest effect on your fitness on the day of the event.

Aerobic Output

Probably the first step in any training program is to work on raising your aerobic output potential. It is simply a matter of strengthening heart and lungs to allow a greater volume of oxygen to reach the muscles. Increasing $\dot{V}_{O2max}$ is the technical way to describe it, and Fig. 12.3 shows how both V_{O2max} itself and the percentage of that maximum that can be used tend to increase with training.

All regular fitness programs emphasize this kind of work, since it is perhaps the best indicator of your physical condition. If you are a runner or have regularly participated in another sport, chances are this is not your limiting factor. If, on the other hand, you tend to get out of breath before your muscles begin to ache and strain, or your normal resting pulse is high and increases rapidly with exercise, you probably need to work most on your aerobic output.

Regularly measure your pulse, either at the wrist or just to the side of the Adam's apple: count for 15 seconds and multiply by four to get BPM (beats per minute) and keep a record of it. Take one daily reading before getting up and one shortly after getting up but before doing any strenuous work each morning. If the latter reading is regularly over 70, or exceeds the first reading just as regularly by more than 7, you almost certainly need a lot of aerobic training to lower it. If, on the other hand, the difference between the two varies greatly from one day to the next you may be suffering from overtraining — see Chapter 6.

As you become more accomplished as a bicyclist, the resting pulse should gradually go down quite a bit. A full first season of training should decrease it to something like 50—60. Values of 35—45 BPM are nothing unusual amongst top cyclists. But don't feel you must get down to that same point, since different people may reach their optimum performance at widely different heart rates.

Aerobic power is increased by doing work at a relatively high aerobic level for continuous periods of at least 20 minutes at least 3 times a week. If it's merely a matter of increasing basic aerobic fitness, training need not necessarily be done by cycling, although that will additionally improve your bicycle performance through other effects as well. This relatively low level in terms of

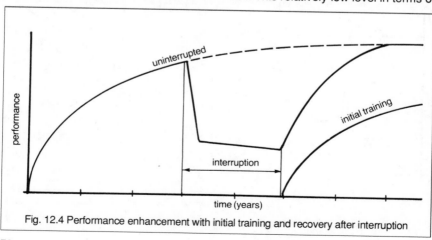
Fig. 12.4 Performance enhancement with initial training and recovery after interruption

duration and frequency may be adequate to reach basic fitness, but doing more work more frequently will prepare you for real training a lot faster. When you start bicycle training seriously, much longer training periods and distances will be required to have any substantial effect at the elevated performance level.

Either way, the aerobic training program will gradually allow the system to bring more oxygen to the muscles at a slower heart rate. Your resting pulse will decrease and you will feel better, because any exertion has less of an impact on your heart rate. The effect of endurance training is most evident on what may be called respiration efficiency: it lowers the number of respirations required to achieve any given volume of air taken in by the lungs. How to go about it in detail will be discussed under the heading *Aerobic Training Methods* below, and in chapters 13 and 14.

It may be interesting to note that the effect of this kind of elementary training (as well as that of several other forms of training), is not lost as easily as it is gained. Once you have reached such a level of physical fitness, very little work may be adequate to maintain it. Besides, after an interruption of up to 5 years, it was found that people who were once fit reached a certain level of fitness much faster than those who were training for the first time in their lives or who had interrupted training for longer periods, as illustrated in Fig. 12.4.

Anaerobic Threshold

That level of exertion beyond which a significant contribution from the anaerobic lactic acid system is required to maintain it is referred to as the anaerobic threshold. You will want to exceed this point at times during your training regimen, because one of the most effective ways to train is pushing this level up higher by exceeding it frequently. In addition, it is assumed that anaerobic capacity itself can also be increased by exercising at such high output levels. Fig. 12.5 shows the effect of anaerobic training on the anaerobic threshold: the outward shift of the curve representing lactic acid concentration in the blood will bring increasingly higher output levels (here represented by %$\dot{V}_{O2max}$) within the range of physical comfort.

There are several objective (though perhaps not conclusive) methods to establish whether the threshold has been exceeded. Since anaerobic work goes hand in hand with the generation of surplus lactic acid, an analysis of the blood for lactic acid concentration will tell whether anaerobic work has been performed. Alternatively, the oxygen consumption can be used as a measure, the underlying assumption being that anaerobic work sets in whenever a certain oxygen consumption rate (itself a guide to the work intensity) is exceeded. The simplest objective method is to measure your actual pulse and to compare it with your base pulse rate, again assuming that this is a reliable measure of the work load.

To complicate things, the anaerobic threshold is not fixed at a given power output level or its corresponding oxygen consumption or heart rate. And as for the

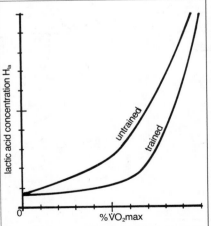

Fig. 12.5 Training effect on aerobic threshold

other method, lactic acid is not the thing you can easily measure anywhere but in a fancy laboratory. Consequently, I favor a seemingly less objective, but ultimately sensitive and conclusive technique of establishing whether you have reached the anaerobic range: it's all in the way you feel.

Your momentary threshold is neither a certain riding speed, nor a certain pulse rate or oxygen intake, nor a certain lactate concentration in the blood. Much less is it the speed that was reached with any of those values some other day. Instead, it is the level where you feel your breathing apparatus can't keep up with the demand for energy and you're hurting. People who concentrate too much on watching their speedometers or measuring their pulse are basing today's assumption on yesterday's performance, which may not be right; it may be either too low or too high. Once you are attuned to your body, you'll always be close to right when you use that as a basis.

Learn to listen to your body. Ride frequent intervals at speeds close to your absolute maximum and establish how it feels. If it doesn't hurt and you recover quickly after an increase in the pace, you probably haven't reached your momen-

tary anaerobic threshold. Eventually, you'll be able to feel when you are there and when you are not. I do suggest you reinforce these subjective findings by taking your pulse occasionally.

Beyond a certain pulse rate you are probably doing anaerobic work, though this figure is also affected by other variables, and changes in the long run as you become more thoroughly trained. Even though this is not the ultimate foolproof indicator, as many people seem to think, it is convenient to establish and reliable enough as long as you correlate the readings to the way you feel from time to time.

Anaerobic Training

Anaerobic training takes place when workouts regularly exceed the anaerobic threshold. Since it overloads the body's systems and raises the lactic acid level in the blood, anaerobic work hurts. After every such workout you will require a recuperation period. As was explained in Chapter 11, regular high-intensity and duration training of any kind will tend to reduce your sensitivity to pain, and consequently anaerobic workouts gradually become less painful, allowing you to use this method of work more and more frequently.

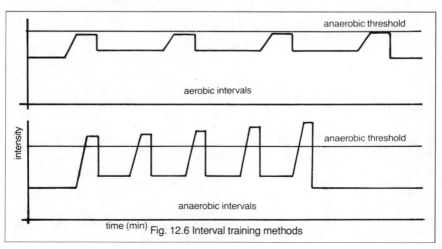

Fig. 12.6 Interval training methods

Generally, anaerobic workouts constitute shortish intervals of very high intensity work during an otherwise aerobic ride. The intervals may constitute either faster pedaling at the same resistance, or a higher resistance at the same pedaling rate. The former are referred to as speed intervals, the latter as power or (more correctly) force intervals. Fig. 12.6 illustrates the effect as it applies to interval training. In other words, these methods simply enable you to train at a higher level of intensity, be that only for short periods.

It cannot be said with certainty whether anaerobic training actually increases your anaerobic capacity, whether it just shifts the anaerobic threshold, or does both. Fact is that virtually all riders make faster progress when their training includes anaerobic work than when it doesn't. Anaerobic training sessions also tax the muscles very much more than aerobic work does. This has the added benefit that the muscle strength is trained more effectively than with most aerobic methods.

Anaerobic training is not for everybody at all times. It is neither suitable for the beginning cyclist in his first season, nor is it wise to take too much of it at any time. It is hard work and should never be done on consecutive days. After avoiding it altogether during the first year, it will be wise to take a break from anaerobic training during a two—three month period in your yearly training schedule, and only get back into doing this kind of work after you have trained aerobically for at least four weeks.

Endurance Training
In Chapter 11, the factors that possibly limit a cyclist's ability to handle long duration work were outlined. Obviously, training to increase endurance must include actual long duration rides, but probably not as many as used to be assumed. If your training schedule includes enough other kinds of workouts, one really long ride a week will be adequate. Preferably, this ride should be at least as long as the toughest event you intend to participate in, and should approximate actual conditions by including more intensive periods of differing duration, ranging from 10 second sprints to 10 minute high speed or high force periods. This is one kind of workout that cannot be done anywhere but on a bicycle on the road: you'd go insane trying to absolve the equivalent of 100 miles on a wind load simulator.

Technique Training
Technique training improves the fluency of movement. One of the most significant effects of initial training is to make the required repetitive movement more fluent and seemingly automatic. When this point is reached, much less energy is wasted than when the legs have to be consciously turned. Technique training is especially required in the initial phase of any training program, and also during the first six weeks of any season if there has been a resting period preceding.

Your pedaling work must become unconscious, yet it will require a lot of very conscious attention to a smooth pedaling style to achieve that. One excellent way is riding a bicycle with a fixed gear (i.e. without a freewheel), using a gear so low that a pedaling rate of at least 80 RPM can be maintained on virtually all terrain encountered. Just the same, training to improve the fluency of movement must not be limited to just pedaling a bicycle, since there are other factors that may hinder your pedaling fluency, but are not easily affected while riding. Stretching and calisthenic exercises, rest, adequate warm-up and post-ride massage all tend to positively influence this factor.

Leg Muscle Training
Since most of the work you will do as a cyclist comes out of the various leg

muscles that were described in some detail in Chapter 14, these are the muscles to develop. This involves more than merely making the muscles bigger and stronger. It is not bulk that counts in cycling — otherwise every accomplished body-builder should be a better cyclist than most top racers. Leg muscle training must mainly be specific, i.e. it must duplicate the speed and the form of movement of actual cycling. Only this will train the muscles to be good at doing exactly the kind of work that will be demanded from them in cycling.

The amount of muscle fiber is the elementary measure of a muscle's potential strength. This can be developed by doing enough cycles of concentric muscle work at a high enough force level. But it is only one of several factors of importance in this respect. The sequence of activity of the various muscles, the contraction speed and the typical range of contraction are all at least as important. Unlike basic strength, these aspects cannot be trained anywhere but on a bicycle — be that on the road or on a windload simulator.

All muscle training exercises should duplicate as closely as possible each of the specific kinds of work that will be demanded in competition. In order to increase sprinting strength, only very fast anaerobic work will do the trick, while aerobic work at a high enough resistance level will improve the kind of muscle strength that is mainly associated with the red slow twitch fibers that are used primarily during aerobic power generation. Don't expect miracles though: if your genetic makeup includes a low proportion of fast twitch fibers, no amount of high intensity work will turn you into an excellent sprinter. You may be flogging a dead horse, so monitor your progress and taper off if you are no longer improving, however hard you work at it. In that case, start developing another aspect of cycling,

and you'll probably improve faster than you had thought possible.

Training of Restraining Muscles
These are the muscles that are not used concentrically during cycling very much, but help by countering forces created with the leg muscles. The arms, shoulders, back and stomach muscles fall in this category. Since they are not used concentrically, they will not get strengthened during cycling, even though they may limit your performance. These muscles can only be strengthened through weight training and calisthenics or other gymnastic exercises. In addition to exercising the muscles for greater strength, stretching and calisthenics may be useful to achieve greater suppleness in these and other muscles.

A basic understanding of which muscle does what and how certain exercises affect a specific muscle will be necessary. Reference to the explanation in Chapter 9 and the specific instructions in Chapter 14 will take care of that. Remember, only the muscles that are contracted will be strengthened: to strengthen the stomach muscles, no amount of body bending will help, unless you pull up forcefully.

Aerobic Training Methods
In this and the following sections, we will describe the basic training methods in common use, starting off with the most common. Aerobic exercises are all those forms of training in which the body is not forced to operate beyond the anaerobic threshold and hence no surplus lactic acid is generated. This group of exercises can include both short and long duration work, both on and off the bike. They are most suitable to increase general aerobic power (if performed close to the anaerobic threshold, even if not for very long periods) and endurance (if continued for a long period of time). The rule of thumb

to establish whether an aerobic exercise is effective is the pulse rate. If anaerobic work is not desired, the pulse, measured in beats per minute, should not exceed the maximum level determined by the following formula:

$$BPM_{max} = 0.85 \times (220 - \text{age in years})$$

For an adequate increase in V_{O2max} and aerobic power, the pulse rate, though remaining below the value calculated above, must exceed the level determined by the following formula:

$$BPM_{min} = 0.75 \times (220 - \text{age in years})$$

During the first five minutes of exercise, the pulse tends to increase and vary quite a bit. Consequently, the pulse should be measured after at least five minutes of exercise.

Anaerobic Training Methods
These include all exercises — again both on and off the bike — in which the surplus lactic acid generating anaerobic system is activated. Their benefit lies in an increase of overall anaerobic capacity and probably in an increased immunity to the pain that causes the lesser athlete to give up. In addition, muscle strength may be increased with this form of work whenever it is more ·geared towards high muscle force than toward high speed work. This kind of training should not be attempted until after a satisfactory basic level of fitness and a smooth riding style have been reached: don't do it in your first season.

Interval Training Methods
These methods are based on the overcompensation effect discussed earlier in this chapter. They include any forms of exercise that include a cyclical increase and subsequent reduction of workload from a lower aerobic base rate of power. Each interval training session consists of a number of repeated exercises. One high output period with one recovery period is referred to as a repetition, while a sequence of perhaps five or more of these repetitions is referred to as one set. A full interval training session may consist of several of these sets, separated by recovery periods.

Interval training may be either aerobic or anaerobic, even though the recovery periods are always aerobic. In anaerobic interval training the high power surges are largely anaerobic, whereas in aerobic interval training the higher load periods are still aerobic and of a longer duration (several minutes, as opposed to less than thirty seconds each). Both techniques lend themselves equally well to cycling on the open road and to work on the wind load simulator or ergometer.

The training effect on muscle condition, staying power, aerobic power, as well as probably anaerobic threshold and anaerobic power (in the case of anaerobic interval work) are quite dramatic. It should be the mainstay of any program for people whose time is limited. This is certainly so once they have reached a basically adequate level of aerobic fitness, staying power and cycling technique through a more varied training program during the first few years.

Force Training Methods
That's a term not used much elsewhere, but I consider it essential to distinguish this general category of training from weight training, which is but one particular form of it. It is nothing but specific muscle training. The muscles are strengthened by being used concentrically at a high force level, whether that is on the bike in sprinting or climbing, or by means of weights or an exercising machine.

Muscles are strengthened on the bike by pushing very hard in a relatively high gear for pure strength. To make the exercise more selective, this form of training should always be combined with periods of higher pedaling rates in gears that can be ridden at 80 RPM or more to achieve a muscle speed training effect.

As discussed in the section *Training of Restraining Muscles*, above, the non-active (i.e. restraining) muscles must be treated differently. Training restraining muscles, such as those of the arms, shoulders, back and stomach, cannot be done on the bike. It must be done in the form of weight training, although various kinds of calisthenic exercises may be equally effective, and both the latter and stretching will improve the general condition of these muscles.

Technique Training Methods
These include any kind of work to improve the fluency and efficiency of movement, both on the road and on the wind load simulator. The latter has the advantage of allowing close observation (use a mirror if you can't round up a competent live observer). Pedaling unconsciously fast and smoothly is what you are trying to achieve, and doing the same very consciously is what will get you there This form of training should be practiced during the first year and again in the early preparation period of each subsequent year.

Control Method Training
This method allows the cyclist to select his training methods and the types of exercises more intelligently. On the basis of a number of standard test exercises, the progress is verified from time to time.

With a stopwatch and a bicycle computer you can thus check whether the methods used to date have helped improve your performance in a certain discipline. If not, it will be time to consider a different method or a different kind of exercise to achieve further improvement.

Other Exercises
This category includes any exercises that can be done in places ranging from your living room to a gym without either a bike or other mechanical aids. These exercises must also be done with some knowledge of what can be achieved and how to do it. These include stretching, calisthenics and breathing exercises, all discussed in Chapter 14.

Personalized Training
Before we shall go on to specific training methods in the next two chapters, let me give you some basic advice. You are the one to do the training and you are the one to decide how to go about it. Perhaps the most serious mistake to make is blindly copying someone else's training schedule or methods. Train to strengthen your weaknesses, but also learn to emphasize the development of those aspects that best exploit your natural inclinations. If you seem to be a good sprinter, there will be no point in wasting hundreds of hours trying to become equally good at long distance work. Instead, it will be better to merely develop your endurance ability to reach the level where you can keep up with the pack, then make the most of your sprinting ability by training that to the utmost.

The other very individual aspect is the total intensity of training you are able to handle. To ride successfully at the level of club riders, you can probably get by admirably with a training schedule that includes less than half the number of hours that are often recommended. You will probably need one long ride each week, but an intelligent use of more intensive training techniques will allow you to minimize the hours spent training to something suitable for a person with a normal social life.

13. On-the-Bike Training Methods

In this chapter we shall finally get down to brass tacks with some practical training procedures. Presented here are those techniques that must be carried out riding your bike on the road. If you have absorbed the preceding chapters, you have most of the knowledge needed to understand the effects each of the techniques here described has on specific aspects of your performance potential.

Any training methods that can be done on the bike have the potential advantage of allowing greater specificity than most other forms of exercises. As explained in Chapter 12, specificity is the quality of training in approaching the actual kind of movements and other characteristics to be developed most closely. It is essential for effective progress to keep this requirement in mind when selecting training methods, whether with regards to speed, pedaling force, terrain type or distance. The other critical consideration is to emphasize a particular element in each training ride. To give an example, pay attention to technique to improve that same aspect.

On-the bike training methods include several broad categories. These can each be divided into a number of distinct exercises, that are each based on the same training principle. In the following sections the various specific exercises within their respective categories shall each be explained. Five broad categories of training methods can be distinguished:

- LSD or aerobic training;
- aerobic interval training;
- anaerobic interval training;
- technique training;
- control method training.

None of these methods alone, nor even all of them together, make a satisfactory comprehensive training program. Even if all your bike training is done on the road, in which case you may be tempted to ignore the advice on off-the-bike training in the next chapter, you should not forget to include several essential supplementary activities that fall outside the preceding list.

In the first place, every strenuous training ride or organized event should be preceded by a low intensity warm-up period of at least 5 minutes, or up to ten minutes in colder weather. This will condition your joints and muscles and activate the enzyme systems that are essential for muscle effectiveness. In addition, some breathing and gymnastic or stretching exercises should be included in any regular training program, as well as massage after hard long distance riding. Refer to Chapter 14 for details of these techniques. And towards completion of the ride, you should cool off or unwind by cycling at a low intensity level for five minutes or more before getting off the bike.

LSD or Aerobic Training

LSD stands for long slow (or steady) distances. Don't take that S for slow too literally: your speed should at least suffice to work up a sweat, even in cold weather. This used to be the staple diet of bicycle racers and fitness seekers alike. It consists of nothing more than riding a considerable distance at a relatively high but aerobic output level. Its effect is an increase in aerobic capacity and endurance, mainly through a training induced increase of the cardio-respiratory capacity and its efficiency.

Done over relatively short distances (20—30 minutes duration), this is basic fitness work. Carried out over longer distances, it is still the aerobic mainstay of most training programs and is particularly useful during the early part of any season. Although the way you feel can be a reliable indicator of the power expended, the heart rate in BPM can be used to determine whether you are working hard enough. Use the following formulas as upper and lower limits. The pulse should be measured after at least five minutes of intensive work (i.e. after at least ten minutes of riding, including five minutes of warm-up):

$$BPM_{min} =$$
$$0{,}75 \times (220 - age\ in\ years)$$
$$BPM_{max} =$$
$$0.85 \times (220 - age\ in\ years)$$

In an elementary fitness training program, the beginning athlete should absolve a twenty minute session of this at least 3 times a week until the rest of his training program has reached the point of including a much greater amount of work. This won't be anything like enough to qualify as endurance training, and is only a fraction of the distances covered later in a more ambitious training program. It is merely the simplest way to reach an aerobic basis from which to prepare for more intensive bicycle training.

To increase aerobic power once this elementary level of cardiorespiratory fitness has been reached, maintain LSD rides on your schedule at least once a week. The distance should be increased gradually until at least once a fortnight your training ride slightly exceeds the longest organized event you intend to participate in. Preferably such a ride should be spiced with small doses of some of the other elements of your training program. Pay close attention to riding style and pedaling rate during these rides. Initially maintain a relatively low gear and gradually raise your pedaling rate until you can spin for hours on end at well in excess of 80 RPM. Only after you have reached that, should you very gradually start choosing slightly higher gears to increase speed and force, while maintaining the same high pedaling rate.

Aerobic Interval Training

This method consists of a relatively long aerobic ride, interrupted repeatedly by periods of increased intensity. During most of the ride your pulse should remain below the lower limit of the formula above, while you should approach the maximum aerobic rate during the intervals. If all is well, the body's tendency to overcompensate after periods of hard work will have an effect similar to the one illustrated in Fig. 12.2 in the preceding chapter. In each subsequent interval, you may be able to work more intensively, leading to a more rapid increase of aerobic power, muscle strength and endurance.

On the bike, aerobic interval training methods include any form of aerobic riding characterized by differentiated speed or intensity. This may range from structured rides, planned out in advance, to occasional speeding in higher gears or faster spins in the same gear, to the accidental changes forced by riding in hilly terrain or in heavy traffic. The latter technique is only recommended for those who have enough traffic sense and experience to be safe in traffic and who have enough self discipline to stay within the aerobic range, even if the next traffic light will turn red on you if you don't speed like the devil. Fartlek is a fancy Scandinavian term for unstructured aerobic interval training.

A 20—30 mile ride like this, consisting of perhaps five faster or tougher repetitions of 1—1.5 miles each, separated by easier periods of 2—3 miles each, will probably provide more effective aerobic training than an LSD ride over twice the distance. Since it is harder to care for proper technique while doing this work, it is not recommended for your first season or the early part of any subsequent season. Later in your racing career, aerobic intervals may gradually replace essentially all LSD work after the first month of each season, except the biweekly long ride.

Anaerobic Interval Training

That's aerobic rides, repeatedly interrupted by very fast or hard intervals. They help increase anaerobic strength, improve sprinting and climbing performance, and raise the anaerobic threshold. To the casual observer this may seem like the same thing as the type described above, but there are some significant differences: the work intervals are shorter and much more intensive, requiring anaerobic output, and the recovery intervals are ridden at a considerably lower intensity. During the work intervals the pulse will rise above the maximum figure suggested by the formula above, and it may be somewhat higher for each subsequent interval.

The first set of intervals must be preceded by a relatively light warm-up ride during at least 10 minutes. Then a number of sets, each consisting of several repetitions is ridden. Each repetition consists of a high intensity effort over a relatively short distance, followed by a recovery period over five or more times that same distance. The repetitions should have increasing and declining lengths, and between sets the heart rate is allowed to return to about 100—110 BPM.

Once you are familiar with the process, there will be no need to check your pulse each time, since you will have developed a feel for your condition. Between consecutive sets the power output level may be reduced by gearing down, so that a high pedaling rate is retained without requiring excessive force. A typical set may consist of five repetitions with efforts of varying length; each session may consist of five or more such sets, separated by periods of moderate aerobic riding.

The length of the efforts is best expressed in crank revolutions, since they are easiest to count. Remember that in a reasonably high racing gear each crank revolution corresponds to about 7—8m (say an average of 25 feet). The intervals must be relatively short, since the anaerobic power would be soon depleted otherwise. Typical effort distances may vary to reflect the kind of riding they are to prepare for, and it is wisest to use both long and short effort sets within your training program.

A typical training program would comprise a number of sets, each consisting of repetitions with efforts of 10, 20, 30, 20, 10 crank revolutions. A program for road racing and time trialing might include longer repetitions. In either case, do not attempt to ride more sets than you can handle feeling fit, because the training effect does not depend on how tired you feel, but on how high the output was, and the output invariably falls off as you become too fatigued.

Anaerobic interval work is a wonderful training technique to strengthen sprinting and climbing power, though it doesn't hurt to include some of it in every training schedule, whatever discipline most suits your talents. Whatever your goal, it is recommended not to do hard interval work (or any other form of anaerobic training involving high muscle forces) the day before or after a tough organized event. In fact, it will be safest never to do it on consecutive days: alternate days with and days without anaerobic interval training.

Commonly, distinction is made between speed intervals and power intervals. The latter is a misnomer for what should correctly be referred to as force intervals. In speed intervals, mainly suited to develop muscle speed and staying power, choose a slightly lower gear and increase the pedaling rate until a distinctly higher speed is reached, at which point a higher gear may again be in order.

Force intervals are good for increasing muscle strength, in addition to general anaerobic power. To do this, choose a slightly higher gear and try to increase the pedaling rate at the same time. With either type of work, drop back to aerobic levels before you are thoroughly exhausted.

Neither of these exercises should be attempted by newcomers. Wait until you have developed a flawless riding style and have absolved at least one year of training. Otherwise, the potential for injury is significant and your riding style may suffer. During the first few months of this kind of work, I'd use speed intervals only, not introducing force intervals until later. If signs of overtraining develop (as outlined in Chapter 6), force intervals should be the first thing to drop from your schedule; if signs persist, refrain from all anaerobic work.

Technique Training

If any form of training is frequently neglected, this is it. Few riders seem to be aware that an improved technique — including both pedaling style and bike handling — can do more for a their overall performance than any kind of training for strength, once a basic level of fitness has been reached. I suggest setting aside at least two fifteen minute portions of your training time each week in which you pay close attention to pedaling, gearing and handling techniques. This is particularly necessary during your first year of serious cycling, but should be kept upin subsequent years too.

Refer to Chapter 3 for the kind of things to pay attention to in technique training. Certainly in the early preparation stage of each new training year the pedaling style should receive close scrutiny. This is best done on a bike with a fixed gear in a lowish gear, selecting light and level terrain for this purpose. For your other technique rides, find different kinds of terrain occasionally, to become familiar with the bike's behavior under widely varied conditions. If at all possible, group rides should also be included, in which you can practice techniques of drafting, or pacing, as well as skills needed for riding close together without accidents.

Control Method Training

This is my term for those procedures that allow you to evaluate your performance and progress. It can make your training more specific and scientific.

The principle is that repeating identical exercises at different times during your training year will give some conclusive answers about the effectiveness of your training procedure, and may suggest on which techniques to concentrate. At the same time, this method may make it clear where your natural abilities and your weaknesses lie.

To carry out control training, identify several stretches of road with particular characteristics: long and short smooth level stretches and climbs of different gradients. Determine some simple landmarks, such as milestones. Try to find several very similar stretches that under neutral conditions take the same time to cover. If at all possible, include at least three of the items on the following list in the trial stretches you select:

* 200m, or 0.1 mile, on level roads;
* 1km, or 0.7 mile, on level roads;
* An 8km, or 5 mile, loop on mainly level terrain;
* A 30km, or 20 mile, loop on mainly level roads;
* A number of short climbs of similar steepness with identical differences in elevation (e.g. 10m, or 30 ft);
* One or more long climbs of similar steepness with identical elevation differences (e.g. 100m, or 300 ft).

At least once every three months, after some light warm-up work, ride two or three of these at your maximum output for the appropriate distance, measuring your time accurately. Keep a systematic record of your times and any peculiarities you noticed during the ride, as well as the way you felt afterwards and your pulse rate during recovery. Summarize this information in the form of a table, which allows you to easily compare results over time.

Evaluate the changes between the results every three months. Whenever significant continuous trends of improvement show up, you may conclude that further improvement is possible by continuing the same or similar training methods. When, on the other hand, little or no improvement is apparent, you are either flogging a dead horse or not training effectively to develop the particular skills needed for that discipline. You have probably reached one of the dips in the set of short-cycle curves shown in Fig. 12.1: it is time to change horses.

Decide on the basis of the preceding chapter whether you should modify your training in one or more points to become more effective. However, it is just possible you have reached a genetically determined limit in a particular discipline. In that case, no type or amount of training will bring much progress. No need to neglect that discipline altogether, but time to concentrate on some other aspect.

If your anaerobic performance in sprinting and climbing is not improving, even after you have tried more intensive training techniques, you may decide that your strengths lie elsewhere. In an event, try not to get yourself in the situation where a fast sprint will be decisive. If, on the other hand, your sprints are fine but long time trial performance does not improve, even with longer and more intensive training techniques, you may use your skills to best advantage by making the most of your anaerobic abilities, letting your companions do most of the work on those long straight stretches, while you take the lead storming a hill to keep your spirits up.

14. Indoor Training Methods

In this chapter, we shall consider the various methods of training that can be carried out without the use of a bicycle on the road. Included are both exercises that are impossible to do on the bike, and methods in which other techniques are used to substitute for riding the bicycle on the road. The former are needed to supplement the training regimen wherever pure bicycle training is not suitable or adequate to develop certain skills, the latter are mainly used when unfavorable factors inhibit bicycle training out of doors.

Calisthenics and Stretching

These forms of exercises in bicycle training comprise a complex of simple movements to loosen joints and increase the flexibility of muscles. Some of these exercises may also help develop muscles that are not adequately used concentrically in cycling to be trainable by riding the bike. In addition, light exercises of this kind can be useful to loosen and warm up before hard training or organized rides. This may achieve an optimal enzyme activity, necessary for maximum muscle performance, as well as minimizing fatigue. Finally, this kind of work may ease recovery after long duration hard riding.

The difference between calisthenics (or gymnastics) and stretching lies in the continuity of movement. Each type has its adherents, and my opinion is that a combination of the two forms is best. Certainly when the weather is cold, stretching will do more harm than good. For that reason I recommend refraining from that kind of exercise outside when the temperatures are low: do calisthenics instead. Even if the air is not cold, your muscles and joints are probably not warm enough when you first start out. Consequently, stretching should always be preceded by some form of warming-up, either cycling, jog-ging or doing calisthenics. Both calisthenics and stretching exercises are not a substitute for bicycling. They merely complement cycling and improve your physical condition. Specifically, these exercises have the following effects:

- Increase movement angles of the joints used in cycling;
- Strengthen muscles that are used isometrically in cycling;
- Condition the muscles to use a larger range of movement between maximum contraction and maximum reach;
- Prevent aches or cramps resulting from tenseness while cycling.

In calisthenics, joints are loosened and muscles conditioned as the body is bent and subsequently stretched in a swinging motion over the greatest joint angle possible (this angle will usually increase significantly with repeated practice)

Of the muscle pairs at any joint, the single muscles that are stretched in calisthenics may be strengthened; however, not as a result of the stretching, but of the subsequent contraction when the joint is straightened forcefully again.

In stretching, joints and muscles are conditioned to extend fully by forcing them statically in an extremely extended or contracted position, which is reached gradually and then held for at least 30 seconds.

On the accompanying pages some useful exercises of both types are depicted in Fig 14.1 and Fig. 14.2. These are selected in part specifically for bicycle training, in part for their general effect on overall physical wellbeing. One 10 minute session every other day will be adequate for most fitness cyclists.

Breathing Exercises

Efficient breathing technique can have a

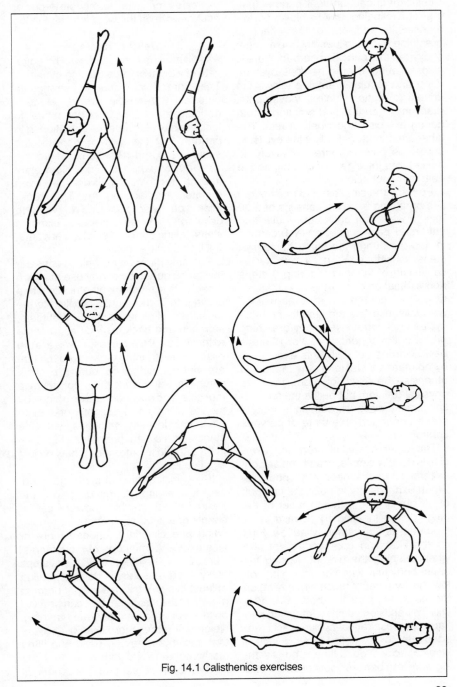

Fig. 14.1 Calisthenics exercises

significant impact on your general feeling of wellbeing and athletic performance. In addition to the effect of breathing depth, influencing the amount of oxygen that can be absorbed, there is also an effect on the nervous system: deep and regular breathing allows the brains to better control movements, reactions, thoughts and emotions, both during exercise and when at rest. The latter effect may well allow the cyclist to divide his powers more effectively, to make more intelligent decisions, and to train more consciously.

Perhaps the simplest and most effective breathing exercise consists of a 20 minute walk at a brisk but regular and unhurried pace, consciously breathing in and out during the same number of steps each time. Start off with cycles consisting of inhalation during 6 steps and exhalation during the next 6 steps. Over the course of several weeks, gradually increase the lengths of these cycles until you are regularly breathing in and out over periods of 9 or 10 steps each. Carried out daily, this exercise is by no means a waste of time that could otherwise be used for more intensive physical training, but builds the foundation for an excellent breathing technique and an unperturbable state of nervous control.

The other essential breathing exercise is equally simple. Breathe in and out several times as deeply as possible. When exhaling, try to push the last puff of air out of the farthest corner of the lungs; when inhaling try to take in as much air as your lungs will allow. First do this standing up, bending forward when pushing the air out, raising the upper body fully when breathing in. Follow this by a set of these when lying on the back, keeping the body relatively still. Two sessions daily, comprising perhaps ten respiration cycles each, are adequate to maximize your effective lung capacity. A good time to do breathing work is in between sets of calisthenic exercises or after a moderate-power bout of work on the wind load simulator.

Weight Training

As you may have noticed, I am no advocate of weight or force training methods. They are intended to strengthen muscles. But muscle strength alone is no indicator of bicycle performance. In fact, the muscles must be conditioned to perform just the kind of work, at the same speed and in the same sequence, as required when cycling. No weight training technique will do that even remotely as effectively. And if you really think you need this kind of work to develop your leg muscles, climbing stairs, taking two or three steps at a time, will be equally effective.

The only muscles for which I consider this technique to be of any use at all are those that are used isometrically when cycling. In particular, this applies to the muscles of the arms, shoulders, stomach and back, as well as to some extent those of the calves. These are the essential restraining muscle groups that are not strengthened during cycling, since isometric work does not develop muscles, and may perhaps be trained by means of selective weight work. Even so, some low-key solutions, such as standing on a slant board (see Fig. 19.3 in Part III) ten minutes a day, may be just as effective.

If you insist, this is how to go about weight training: Depending on the desired effect (fast high-power work for sprints or sustained strength for regular riding and climbing), choose more or less explosive methods of movements. Pure force training, which develops bulky short muscles, is done repeating at least five times with a weight or force of 80% of the maximum that can be lifted once. For more moderate training, weights or forces more like 50—60% of that maximum may be used and lifted more frequently. Do your weight training in the form of several brief periods preceded and separated by light exercises, such as low- intensity aerobic work on the wind load simulator.

Fig. 14.3 shows some of the useful weight exercises to strengthen restraining muscles. What really counts should be concentric force training, and that is quite possible without any fancy gadgets: simple calisthenic exercises such as push-ups, sit-ups, rowing and

torso raising will probably work just as well and can be done anywhere without any gadgetry. Either way, three sessions a week, depending in length on your available time will generally be adequate.

Roller Training
The old fashioned way of indoor training for is with the bicycle placed on a set of

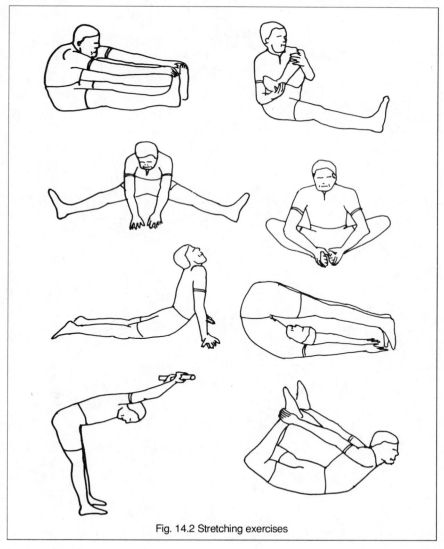

Fig. 14.2 Stretching exercises

rollers. It's hard to balance the bike at first, but it has its charm once you get used to it. Whether it does you any good remains to be seen. The rollers provide virtually no resistance, which allows you to pedal without much effort at the maximum pedaling rate your body will be able to handle. That is probably the only use for this form of exercise: it allows you to work on increasing your maximum pedaling rate, which is essential for beginners and useful for any cyclist after a longer layoff.

Ergometer Training

An ergometer is a kind of stationary pedaling device with a big flywheel and a variable resistance. Changing the

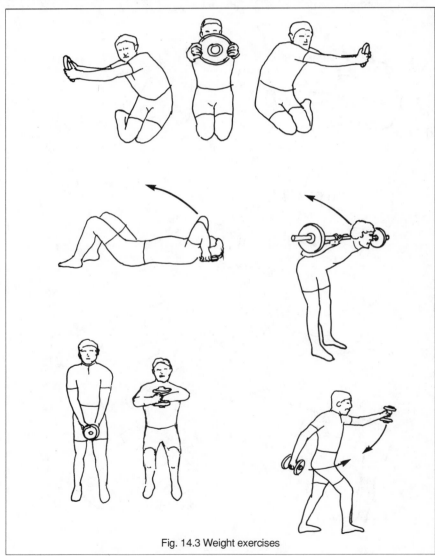

Fig. 14.3 Weight exercises

resistance and adjusting your pedaling rate allows variations in power and apparent speed, comparable to differences during actual cycling. That's a big improvement over the roller training described above, but it's not the last word in stationary bicycle training. In the first place, all bicycle ergometers are hopelessly uncomfortable, having been designed for (and by) those sedentary types who are more familiar with armchairs than with bicycles. More importantly, the kind of resistance offered does not allow you to simulate actual riding situations, where the required power increases exponentially with the speed, due to air resistance. Finally, it is impossible to cool the rider on a conventional ergometer.

Wind Load Simulator Training

This equipment, also referred to as turbo-trainer, is the answer to a maiden's prayer. It overcomes the inadequacies of ergometers on the one hand and of rollers on the other hand. Here the bike can be attached to a structure on top of a set of rollers that drive a set of wind turbine wheels (or nowadays often electric devices that give the same kind of variable drag that increases with speed). As the speed of the rear wheel increases, either due to faster pedaling in the same gear or to the selection of a higher gear at the same pedaling rate, the air resistance increases exponentially, resulting in the drastic increase in required power typical of cycling at higher speeds under real-world conditions.

Several of these devices can be equipped with a system of air ducts to guide the air that is scooped up by the turbines to discharge a stream of cooling air at the rider's face and chest, which is surprisingly effective. The wind load simulator, especially when equipped with such a cooling system, combines the best possible simulation of real world cycling conditions, with the advantage of being stationary, allowing close monitoring and use under conditions unfavorable to riding the bike.

Mounting an electronic speedometer with additional functions for pedaling speed and pulse rate monitoring provides you with the ultimate in stationary training and monitoring equipment: an exercise physiology lab of your own. Referring to the preceding chapters will allow you to make sensible training decisions, to be implemented on the wind load simulator as well.

Virtually every one of the training techniques described in Chapter 13 for cycling on the road can also be carried out quite satisfactorily on the wind load simulator. Excepted are only those technique elements that relate to the bicycle's handling. You can ride a moderate gear and speed for a protracted aerobic exercise. You can spin frantically in a low gear to improve your pedaling rate, or you may carefully observe your pedaling style at different speeds and power levels. You can simulate sprints and climbs and you can carry out various types of interval training for more effective high intensity aerobic and anaerobic workouts.

The windload simulator is the ideal tool of control method training. The situation is not so strongly affected by extraneous influences and it is easier to monitor and record the results in terms of minutes and seconds. The effects of the work on your body can also be observed and recorded more easily.

Set up a schedule of wind load simulator exercises that correspond more or less to the items on the list from Chapter 13. Carry these (or at least the ones that seem relevant to your training goals) out once every three months, keeping close track of progress. With the modern programmable trainer, it is simple to select a program that gives you the load variations you need.

Don't forget to do the most important part: evaluate the changes and developments over time as a function of your training methods, modifying your techniques as dictated by that evaluation. Train your weak points only as much as seems justified by a continuing improvement.

Don't start out hard without warm-up and don't break off training immediately after an anaerobic or otherwise high intensity exercise, but continue work at a reduced output level for several minutes before stopping. Also observe the rule that both intensive anaerobic workouts involving high muscle forces and extremely long training periods should be avoided on consecutive days, as they should be on days immediately preceding or following a tough organized ride.

Cyclo-Computers

Take a windload simulator and a cyclist's brains, then replace the latter by a computer, and you have what is referred to as a cyclo-computer these days. It's the ultimate training tool, according to most of my colleagues. I agree only partly: it applies only as long as you use it as a tool rather than becoming it's slave.

Cyclo-computers can be programmed to give you the ride you select on this latest electronically controlled edition of the humble turbo-trainer. But only an intelligent decision what kind of ride you want to achieve your consciously selected training goals makes this instrument a tool rather than making you a slave. Only too often, the opposite is the case. Use it wisely, and you can set up a very satisfactory indoor training schedule on the lines of what was described here for cycling on the road in the preceding chapter or for turbo-trainer work in the present one.

Massage

Though it may not appear to be a training practice, massage has long been recognized as a suitable way of improving both performance and training progress, as well as preventing cramps and injuries. In the context of this book, the most useful remarks on massage will be some guidelines for self- administration. It's nice if you have a specialist do it for you, but you can do it yourself quite effectively. Since only you can tell how you really feel, this may well be the most effective method anyway.

The most probable justification for massage is the encouragement it provides for the enzyme and blood circulation systems local to the muscles. Another theory holds that in hard, repeated muscle exercise, small fissures are formed and wastes (mainly lactates) accumulate in these fissures

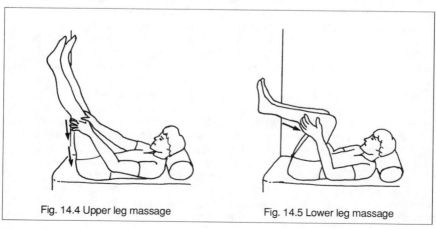

Fig. 14.4 Upper leg massage   Fig. 14.5 Lower leg massage

within the muscle. Massage is then presumed to encourage the removal of these wastes and to reinstitute a complete flow of blood that can take care of full recovery.

Whatever the merits of either theory, in practice massage works well and is recommended specifically after particularly long or hard rides. It prevents the 'day after' muscle aches and allows more effective training, even if it is not administered immediately after a hard century ride or training session.

Procedure for Self-Massage
1. Take a shower or merely wash the legs in warm (but not hot) water, and dry them thoroughly. There is no real need to use massage oil.
2. Lie comfortably on your back, at such a distance from the wall that you can stretch your legs above you as shown in Fig. 14.4.
3. Grab the middle of one of the thighs firmly with both hands, surrounding the muscle bundles; rub forcefully with long, even strokes

down from that point towards the hip. Continue this for about one minute.
4. Now do the same for the section of the thigh from the knee down to the location just beyond where you started under point 3. Apply similar regular strokes, continuing for about one minute.
5. Repeat the work covered in points 3 and 4 for the other thigh.
6. Move back from the wall to take the position shown in Fig. 14.5, with the knees bent and the lower leg horizontally.
7. Carry out a similar massage of the lower legs, working towards the knees, as described in points 3—5 for the thighs.
8. Briefly massage the muscles of lower and upper legs with about ten long strokes over their entire length.

Afterwards, rest a few minutes, lying on your back with the legs raised. Finally, wash and dry your legs.

15. Your Personal Training Plan

In this chapter, you will be shown how to put together an individual and systematic schedule for all your fitness and condition training. Only such a tailor-made personal plan will allow you to train really effectively. Based on your knowledge of the various training methods, as well as the assessment of training goals and personal strengths, keeping in mind the time you have available, you should be able to decide which methods and techniques to employ and how much time to devote to each.

This training plan should be broken down into four stages, corresponding to different time horizons. You will need a long range plan for your active cycling life, an annual one for the current or next year, an intermediate range plan for any one of the periods of 2—5 months each into which the year is divided, and finally a weekly plan that summarizes your daily training routines in detail. Each of these plans must be constantly under consideration for review at time intervals appropriate to their particular time horizons.

No book can give you a ready made plan like this. Copying the plan structured by famous coach A for successful racer B is probably the worst thing you can ever do. Coach A has determined that plan on the basis of the strengths, needs and potentials offered by that particular racer, whom he knows intimately. Had he known you as well, he might have made up an equally suitable plan for you, but it would look quite different, since your strengths, needs and potentials are not the same. The best I can do is show you how such a schedule may be structured and how to go about designing one that suits you personally.

Even so, it will take time. Don't expect to sit down one evening with pen and paper and draw up your training plan, let alone do that before you start riding. And whatever you may have been led to believe elsewhere, a computer won't do this any faster or more reliably. Instead, you must see the structure of your training plan as a growing organism that slowly incubates, develops and matures. Above all, it should be constantly adapted and revised, as you evaluate the results of your training methods to date, reflected by both actual performance and the control methods described in the preceding chapters 13 and 14.

Though the training plan will vary from one individual to the next, I do not recommend emphasizing just one discipline or the other during the year. Try to be an all-round cyclist — one who can handle long trips alone as well as group riding, hill climbing as well as fast sprints. You may be better at the one than at the other, and developing your specific skills to maximum advantage will be useful. Yet you must master all skills adequately if you want to be a really competent cyclist.

Keeping Track

Whatever plan you follow, don't just cycle, but also learn from your experience. Do that by keeping a training log, i.e. a diary in which you write for each day what kind of training you did, emphasizing also the way you felt afterwards and the effect particular routines seemed to have on both your subsequent performance and general condition.

Make the training log systematic by assigning a double-page spread to each week, and using certain colors for particularly important entries. It is not my intention to tell you just how to set up and fill out your personal training log. I merely want to encourage you to do it and to keep it up. And once you have it, refer to it frequently in order to expand your knowledge of your own body and its way of growing fitter.

The Long Range Plan

Your overall or long range plan should be the most informal one of the four. Perhaps it consists of no more than a handwritten list, stating for each year what you consider significant. It will cover a period of at least several years — your bicycling life as you expect it to develop over time. This plan should be re-evaluated about once a year, as you consider your progress and expectations at the end of the season.

It should not go into any great details about the training techniques you intend to apply. Instead, it should generalize your goals and give a rough outline of the ways you feel they may be reached. Break up the plan by years, indicating for each year what you intend to achieve, in what kind of events you intend to participate, and how intensively you will occupy yourself with particular training disciplines during that year. Before drawing up or revising this plan, consider especially the following questions:

- How important will the sport be in your life — both in the next few years and in the remote future?
- How much time will you have available during the various stages of your active cycling life for training and participation?
- What are your particular strong points and weaknesses, and how can they be exploited and down-played, respectively?
- What is the risk involved to your lifestyle and career plans if you have perhaps decided upon a plan that cannot be carried through?

All aspects of this plan will be subject to change once you are getting more and more involved in the sport. Just the same, for most people the initial aims can be maintained if chosen realistically. Decide on your primary goals in simple terms, which may be anything from 'stay fit until old age', 'participate in century rides', 'get involved in long dis-tance events' to 'become a champion bicycle racer'. Needless to say, those with the latter goal will be more likely to revise their plan downward sooner or later.

At this stage also determine on which type of cycling you will want to concentrate. If you venture beyond recreational fitness cycling and consider racing, there are many different disciplines: road criterium racing, time trials, track racing, cyclo-cross and mountain bike competition.

Next, determine what it will take to reach your goals. That may be anything from a modest weekly pensum of riding to many years' cruel training, or moving to a part of the country where your chosen discipline can be developed more effectively. Before proceeding, consider once more whether it's worth the trouble and what will happen if you're not quite as successful as you had expected.

After all, if you are very ambitious, chances are that you soon discover your goals were unrealistic. If you make drastic changes to your life pattern to accommodate those goals, these can not easily be corrected. It may be better to revise your goals to match the possibilities than it is to try it the other way round. If you should turn out to be that one in a million who can rise to the top quickly, it will soon enough show, at which time it will be early enough to take such drastic steps.

The Annual Plan

Your annual training plan covers the next or present year, divided up over preparation, training, participation and rest or recovery periods. It can be revised at any time during the year, but might best be kept intact as much as possible. If you find it doesn't work as well as you had hoped, it may still not be wise to change horses in mid stream. Instead, adjust next year's schedule to reflect your experiences. Try to get a clear understanding of the way this schedule affects your condition, your lifestyle and your performance, so you will be able to determine what to do differently next year.

It is customary to build up the yearly training plan in the form of four distinct periods, varying in length from two to five months. Neither the terms used for the various stages, nor the exact time periods allotted to each are sacrosanct. However, in most cases the values given here will be appropriate. For most cyclists anywhere in the Northern hemisphere, the year may perhaps best be divided up roughly as follows, keeping in mind that some of these periods may overlap the given dates by several weeks and that the participation in wintertime competition (e.g. cyclocross) may force a shift in these periods.

*Preparation Period
(January—February)*
Before the start of the next training season, this is the period to work on general aerobic condition, basic pedaling technique and perhaps muscle strength. If you take up serious cycling for the first time, it is the kind of training to start with and to keep up much longer, even if the time of year is a different one. The emphasis should be on aerobic rides in lowish gears, paying attention to pedaling rate and style as well as breathing technique. Riding should preferably be done on the road, though the windload simulator or ergometer may be substituted if conditions don't allow riding outside. In addition, you will need to do light calisthenics, stretching and breathing exercises.

Development Period (March—April)
This is the main training period as far as developing strength, speed and endurance is concerned. Gradually, you should introduce more aerobic and (in later years) anaerobic interval training. Start control method training at this time, to monitor your progress. More and

more, you should introduce distances and exercises that are similar in speed and variation to the kind of riding you intend to do later in the year.

Participation Period (May—October)
If you get into racing, this would be the competition period. If you don't, it will be the time most organized rides are offered. Though in many parts of the world you may not be able to participate in organized or sanctioned events as frequently, you will probably do best to adhere to a schedule that simulates the work done by somebody who participates in a major event each week. If you can't participate in real ones, at least do something that simulates structured riding conditions on those days. The rest of the program can perhaps be relaxed a little, but concentrate more and more on the particular discipline in which you perform best. Work towards a climax to gradually peak around the time of the most important major events towards the end of the season.

*Resting Period
(November—December)*
No need to take the word 'resting' too literally, but this is a time to ease off on the amount of training work. Though I feel it is best to continue cycling, many people purposely lie low or change to other forms of exercise. Whatever sport you do, keep it relatively light, avoiding really exhausting work, whether in terms of duration or speed and power. It may also be the time to start working on dietary weight control, if you found you were carrying too much body fat during the season. It is an excellent period to evaluate your performance and the effect of your training schedule so far, talking to others and comparing notes. At the same time, you may read up on the physiological findings related to the sport, as published in the cycling periodicals. This allows you to get more familiar with training and riding methods in general and with your chosen sport in

particular.

The Intermediate Range Plan

This is the schedule for shorter time spans within the various periods just described. These sub-periods may range in length from three weeks to two months. With the exception of the resting period, divide each of the main periods into three parts of unequal lengths.

The short first part is used to introduce and gradually increase the kind of exercises characteristic for that main period. The middle and longest part should emphasize clearly the kind of work to which this period is mainly devoted. In the final part you may intensify your efforts to come to a distinct peak in performance (in the case of the participation period) or gradually start a transition to the next period by introducing features characteristic for it.

The Weekly Plan

Each of the intermediate range periods may be broken up into minor periods of one week each. Within any one of the intermediate range periods the schedule for each week may generally be quite similar, though they will fluctuate in terms of intensity from one week to the next. Obviously, the longest sub-period (the middle part of the participation period) will be most similar over the greatest number of weeks. Yet you should also consider whether any shift of emphasis may be desirable within such a period.

Divide each week up into the seven days, and the days according to your available time. You may not often have uninterrupted blocks of time available for four-hour training rides. This will force you to divide up your time, and intensify the exercises you do in each of the available time blocks. Allocate your time wisely: for example, don't waste valuable winter daylight hours grinding away on a wind load simulator or doing weight training, when you could be out riding the bike, which is so much harder when it is dark and cold.

No need to be guided by the number of hours spent working out by some of the top racers, who have little else to do. Actually, these athletes might perhaps do well to reduce their training workload too. Especially in the participation season, the *training intensity* per training ride is more important than the number of hours spent in the saddle. The same goes for other forms of training. Train consciously and intensively, rather than in drudgery. Of course, you must still try to get some rides in that are quite similar in length and terrain type to the hardest events you will be participating in, in order to satisfy the need for training specificity.

Generally, the schedule during any one sub-period will stay similar from one week to the next. On the other hand, there will be significant differences between weeks in one period and weeks in a different main training period. Consult the preceding guidelines to determine what to emphasize during each of the main periods of your training season, and keep your own preferences and limitations in mind.

Specific Training Schedules

It will obviously be impossible for me to lay out detailed weekly schedules for every week of the year, if only because I don't know you or your personal needs. All I can do is tell you what to consider and give you an illustrative example, not meant to be copied, but to be used for inspiration — examples of what such schedules might con tain.

In the sections that follow, I shall include both schedules for beginning and advanced fitness riders, and a typical schedule for the main sub-period within the participation period. of an ambitious rider. The first example is suitable for the person who wants to get and stay fit, but without any athletic ambition

Basic Fitness Schedule

Sunday:
Event day: Participate in an organized ride of 30 miles or more, preceded by warmup and do some breathing and calisthenics or stretching, perhaps concluded by a light massage.

Monday:
Rest day: Breathing and stretching and/or calisthenics only. Or go for a relaxing walk or short bike ride.

Tuesday:
Rest day: Same as Monday.

Wednesday:
Mid-week training day. 20 mile ride with intervals, again combined with warmup and cooling down, as well as breathing, stretching and/or calisthenics and perhaps massage.

Thursday:
Rest day: Same as Monday.

Friday:
Rest day: Same as Monday.

Saturday:
End-of-week training day. Either participate in another organized ride of 30 miles or more or do a similar ride.

First-Time Century Schedule

This schedule is of course not limited to people preparing for just this distance of 100 miles only. Instead, it is intended for the person who wants to build up enough strength and endurance to participate in one major event over a long duration — an event much tougher than what he or she is used to to date. Here it's a matter of building up strength over a longer period, starting out at the level of the person who follows the basic fitness plan, gradually increasing the intensity and the distance of training. It can be done over a two month period, going about it as follows:

First week:
Increase number of training days from three to four (e.g Saturday, Sunday, Tuesday and Thursday, riding a total of 70—80 miles in the week.

Second—fourth week:
Gradually increase the distance of the Sunday or Saturday ride and the intensity of the mid-week rides. In the fourth week, you should be riding a total of 100—120 miles and include aerobic intervals in the mid-week rides.

Fifth—sixth week:
Increase the length of the Saturday or Sunday ride to a level about 80% of the big event. Add anaerobic interval work (e.g. a few sprints or fast hill climbs), followed by recovery. Total weekly distance should be 1.2— 1.5 times the distance of the big event by the end of the sixth week.

Seventh—eighth week:
Increase the length of the Saturday or Sunday ride to the equivalent of that of the big ride. Continue the weekday rides as before.

Last week before the event:
Do a hard session early in the week and relax a little for the rest of the week. Cut the distances of the Thursday and pre-event day session (i.e. Saturday if the big ride is on the Sunday) to about 20 miles of easy riding. Warm up during the first ten minutes of the big ride or — better yet — ride at a relaxed pace for about that long before the event starts, so you are ready to follow the pace when others set it.

Hard Training Schedule

The third example is for the more ambitious rider, whose schedule allows enough time to approach the training regimen of a moderately interested bicycle racer. Here I summarize the regular weekly training schedule for such a rider during the participation season. Build up to this level of intensity in the early season by increasing the work load from the basic fitness level schedule to the first-time century level in the first two examples. After this you should be ready for the following regimen.

Sunday:
Event day: Participate in an organized century or similar event or a simulated one in the form of repetition and interval rides, including some control work; in addition, do only light aerobic warm-up, stretching, breathing and massage.

Monday:
Rest day: Calisthenics or stretching, breathing and either no cycling at all or some light aerobic work.

Tuesday:
Duration training day: An LSD ride of at least the length of your longest events, as well as some of the other elements of your training program.

Wednesday:
Light training day: Light aerobic rides with aerobic interval work, in addition to smaller volumes of the various other elements.

Thursday:
Hard training day: Fast aerobic and anaerobic interval work over a long distance, including some of the other elements.

Friday:
Intermediate training day: Similar to Tuesday but over a shorter distance.

Saturday:
Light training day: Similar to Wednesday.

Some riders respond more positively to a program in which the intermediate training day precedes the event day. This is the case when the compensation effect outweighs the recovery effect for a particular athlete after a particular workload. Experiment a little by comparing both your results and the way you feel when following the above schedule with those when you have reversed the programs for Friday and Saturday.

Remember that this is really merely an example, valid at best only for one period for some riders. It's a reasonable way to show how such a schedule may be built up, but it is not intended to be strictly adhered to. Perhaps it's a good starting point, but you must actively experiment and think about ways to modify the schedule that suits your possibilities and needs, leading to maximum improvement of your performance. That may take several months, but if you work on it consciously and intelligently, you will be able to devise the optimal training plan to suit your personal needs.

Don't forget that you are not in this for performance alone. To keep fit, you only need to follow the more modest basic fitness schedule. If you don't feel like training like a racer, perhaps it is just as much fun and satisfaction to merely stay fit, doing what you enjoy at the pace that suits you best.

Part III – Know Your Equipment

16. Selecting a Bicycle

In the chapters of this third part, we will cover the equipment. First you will be shown how to go about selecting a bike that is most suited to your purpose, followed in subsequent chapters by a presentation of the various individual bike components and other equipment used in cycling for fitness.

Of course, you probably already have a bike, and there is nothing wrong with using the one you have. Or you may have gone out to a bike shop once you had decided to start cycling for fitness and bought a new bike for the occasion. Nothing wrong with that either: use that bike and it will probably serve you admirably.

But if you were smart or frugal enough to buy this cheap book before splurging on an expensive bike, you will not be disappointed either. Here's some useful advice on buying one. It will be followed in the next two chapters by some words of wisdom about the various parts of the bicycle, so you can be familiar enough with the machine to get the best use out of it.

Parts of the Bicycle

Below, I shall briefly introduce various kinds of bicycles. But let's concentrate on what all have in common first. After all, there are more things the various models share than those that separate them.

Fig. 16.1 illustrates the most important parts of any bicycle. Although a typical racing bike is illustrated, virtually all parts shown will be found on all other bicycles too, even though they may in some cases look different in some details.

The smartest way to look at your bike is by considering the various functional groups, which each comprise several related components. Thus, I like to consider the following functional groups of bicycle components and systems:

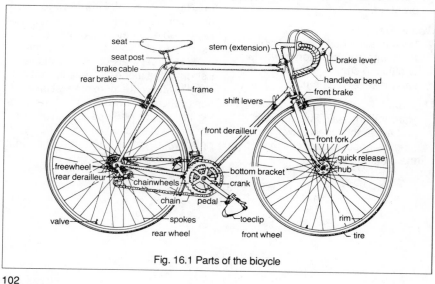

Fig. 16.1 Parts of the bicycle

- the frame;
- the steering system;
- saddle and seatpost;
- the wheels;
- the drivetrain;
- the gearing system;
- the brakes;
- accessories.

In the sections that follow, I shall briefly describe each of these component groups.

The Frame

The frame is the bike's backbone. It is the tubular structure to which all the other components are attached. Full details of the frame, together with information about the steering system and the saddle, will be found in Chapter 17.

The Steering System

The bicycle is steered and — more importantly — balanced, by means of the parts of the steering system. This system comprises the front fork, in which the front wheel is installed and which is pivoted in the front of the frame, as well as the handlebars with the stem that connects them to the fork, and the headset bearings which allow the entire assembly to turn relative to the frame.

Saddle and Seatpost

The bike's seat or saddle is mounted on a tubular section called seatpost. The height of the saddle is adjusted by lowering or raising the seatpost, as it is clamped in the frame's seat tube. The angle and forward position of the saddle are also adjustable, this time by means of an adjustment mechanism integrated in the top of the seat post.

The Wheels

Perhaps the biggest difference between the various types of bicycles is in the wheels: skinny, light ones for racing bikes, fat chunky ones for mountain bikes, heavy ones for utility bikes, small ones for folders and some other less common types. Each wheel consists of a central hub that rotates on ball bearings around the axle mounted in the frame, a rim with a tire mounted on it, and finally a network of spokes that connects the rim to the hub.

The Drivetrain

The set of components that transmits the rider's effort to the rear wheel is referred to as the drivetrain. These parts include the bottom bracket in which the crank spindle rotates on ball bearings, the cranks with the chainrings mounted on the RH one, the pedals, the chain, and the freewheel mechanism with sprockets, or cogs, mounted on the rear wheel hub.

The Gearing System

On virtually all bicycles used today, the gearing, used to adjust the ratio between pedaling speed and riding speed, is taken care of by means of derailleurs. These mechanisms are operated from shift levers and move the chain onto the appropriate combination of chainwheel and sprocket.

The Brakes

Operated by hand levers via flexible bowden cables, the brakes on virtually all modern bicycles squeeze together against the sides of the wheel rims to stop or slow down the wheels and the bike.

Accessories

Mostly, bikes ridden for fitness are devoid of accessories. A few are useful, though: pump, lock, water bottle, and speedometer (usually referred to as bicycle computer). When riding in the rainy and dark season, fenders (or mud guards) and lighting equipment are recommended.

Bicycle Types

Here is a brief summary of the most common bicycle types that lend themselves well to our purpose. Though almost any bike can be used after a fashion, only a limited number of models seem to be in favor with sports riders and will be discussed here.

Racing Bike

The thoroughbred racing bike is a light and rather fragile machine. Shown in Fig. 16.2, it has 12- or 14-speed derailleur gearing, very narrow tires and drop handlebars. It usually weighs in at less than 10kg (22 lbs) and lends itself very well for riding for fitness, especially if you mainly ride on well paved roads.

Triathlon or Sports Bike

This is a simpler version of the racing bike and even more suitable for our purpose. Hard to distinguish, it is generally made with slightly less sophisticated parts and often has more wide-range gearing and a less rigid geometry. The weight is perhaps two or three lbs more than a real racing bike of the same size.

Mountain Bike

Shown in Fig. 16.3, this is the most popular bike sold these days. Originally intended for off-road use, it is also used to advantage on regular roads and city streets. Its thick tires, flat handlebars, powerful brakes and wide-range gearing make it an excellent bike for people who don't feel immediately at ease on a racing or triathlon bike. The weight is usually around 12—14kg (27—30 lbs). Don't overlook the off-road option, since riding cross- country riding is superb for fitness training, especially in the winter season.

Hybrid

Take a mountain bike and install slightly lighter tires, less extremely wide-range gearing and also otherwise make it more suitable for mixed use. You have a hybrid. Quite a nice bike for city use and also very suitable for all less confident riders who don't feel at ease on the true racing bike. Typical weight about 12kg (26—28 lbs).

Touring Bike

A real touring bike looks like a racing bike with luggage racks (carriers) and sometimes fenders (mud guards). There are more differences: heavier gauge materials, more generous clearances, wider tires, the kind of brakes used on a mountain bike and wide-range gearing. These bikes typically weigh about the same as a mountain bike.

Other Models

Yes, though you'll rarely see them used for fitness cycling, there are other bikes as well. They range from utility bikes to three-speeds, from folders to recliners, from tricycles and replicas of ancient machines to futuristic enclosed pedal-driven space capsules. Interesting, but mostly less practical for everyday use.

Bicycle Manufacturers

Most bicycles sold these days are made by major manufacturers. Although there still is a domestic bicycle industry in the US, the vast majority of quality bikes sold through the specialized bicycle

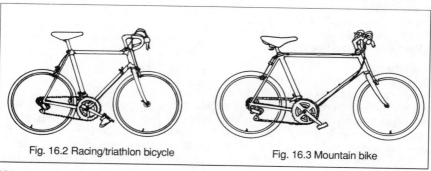

Fig. 16.2 Racing/triathlon bicycle

Fig. 16.3 Mountain bike

trade are imported these days. Most domestically made bikes are the low end mass products sold through non-specialized outlets. Even those major US companies that do sell through the bike trade import most of their products from places like Taiwan, South Korea and Japan. However, several of these manufacturers, such as Trek, Cannondale and Schwinn, still make several top line models in their own US factories.

In addition to these American firms and a number of East Asian manufacturers, the Europeans are not quite dead, although even some of the bikes with European names may well be made elsewhere, particularly if they are less than horribly expensive.

On bikes from many different manufacturers, even custom-built machines, you will find the same frame tubes, brakes, gears, tires, handlebars and a hundred other parts that all come from one of a limited number of manufac-

turers who specialize in those particular items.

Not all parts made by the same firm are of the same quality. A maker of brakes, for instance, may have half a dozen or more different models, ranging in price, type, size and quality from one end of the scale to the other. It will be impossible to give you very detailed information indicating which make and model of any part will be better than other ones, if only because manufacturers change their product specifications and designations from time to time. Instead, I shall explain which general types are suitable and what to look for to make sure you are getting a satisfactory product.

Women's Bikes
Many women have particular difficulties getting a bike to fit them properly. That is due to the manufacturers' desire to standardize. They provide off-the-peg

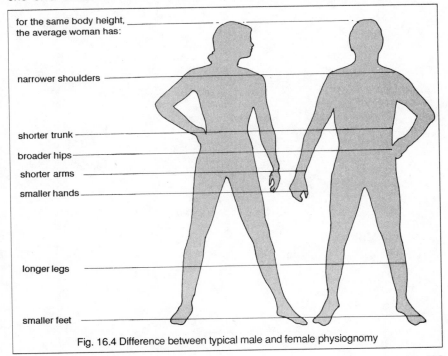

for the same body height, the average woman has:

narrower shoulders

shorter trunk

broader hips

shorter arms

smaller hands

longer legs

smaller feet

Fig. 16.4 Difference between typical male and female physiognomy

frames to fit the averagely proportioned male. However, typically, the woman has different proportions that don't match this scheme. Their legs tend to be longer in relation to trunk and arms. Their arms tend to be weaker and their hips are generylla heavier.

At least one female American manufacturer (Georgina Terry) offers a special series of bikes that are right for the averagely proportioned woman, based on a design pioneered by frame builder Bill Boston. Very fine machines, that are available in many of the more sophisticated bike shops around the country. In addition, some of the major manufacturers now produce similar bikes for women, though they are still not as readily available as women's special needs would suggest.

17. Frame, Steering and Saddle

In the present chapter and the one that follows, you will be shown enough about your bike's major components to ride, handle and maintain the bike most effectively. Yes, you can ride without knowing all the technical ins and outs, but it helps to be informed about the most general concepts. Here we will deal only with the bicycle's backbone: its frame with the steering system and saddle. In the next chapter we'll consider the many components installed on every bike, such as wheels, drivetrain, gears and brakes.

Of necessity, all this will involve some rather basic explanations and definitions of terminology, in addition to specific advice about bicycles and their components. Especially the former is required reading for those who are not fully familiar with the details of the bicycle. Others may be tempted to skip these chapters, assuming they contain nothing new.

Yet even these readers would do well to take this material to heart, since it contains quite a bit of information that will help you select bike and components and to spot what is wrong if your bike doesn't perform the way it should. Furthermore, it will be helpful to at least check the illustrations and their labels, so you become familiar with the terms I shall be using to identify parts of the bike

throughout the book. Often some of these things are called by different names in different parts of the world and indeed by different people in the same area. Thus, confusion can only be avoided if we agree on the terminology that will be used elsewhere in this book.

The Frame

The bicycle's frame, shown in Fig. 17.1, is its biggest single component. It consists of the main frame, built up of relatively large diameter tubes, and the rear triangle, consisting of double sets of tubes with smaller diameters. The main frame is made up of top tube, down tube, seat tube and head tube. The pairs of tubes that form the rear triangle are called seat stays and chain stays, respectively.

On most bikes, the large diameter tubes of the main frame are joined by means of parts referred to as lugs. The seat lug, which connects seat tube and top tube, is slotted in the back, allowing it to clamp around the saddle there. The lug that connects down tube and seat tube is called bottom bracket or chain hanger and accommodates the bearings for the crankset. The two forward lugs, connecting the head tube to down tube and top tube, respectively, are called head lugs and hold the bearings

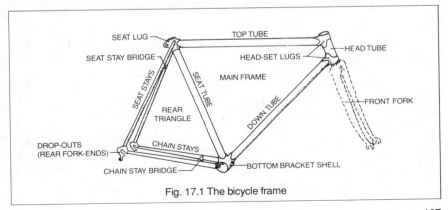

Fig. 17.1 The bicycle frame

of the bike's steering system. Fig. 17.2 shows the difference between typical lugged and lugless frame joints.

The rear triangle's pairs of seat and chain stays each come together in flat plates, referred to as drop-outs or (rear) fork- ends, in which the rear wheel is installed. At the top, the seat stays are attached to the seat lug, while the chain stays run to the bottom bracket. The pairs of these stays are each stiffened by means of short transverse tubular bridge pieces.

Materials, Strength and Rigidity

Although some manufacturers offer very attractive bikes with frames made of aluminum alloy tubing, welded or bonded together with or without lugs, most bikes are still made with more traditional materials: various qualities of steel. On cheap bikes, the frame is made of simple carbon steel tubes that must have significant wall thicknesses (about 1.4 mm) to give adequate strength. This results in a rather heavy and 'dead' bike.

For more expensive machines, strong steel alloys are used. These alloys contain small percentages of other materials, such as chrome, molybdenum and manganese. Generally, their strength is further increased through the tube forming operation. Due to these materials' greater inherent strength, the

resulting frame is strong enough even when the tube wall thickness is much smaller. On the quality frames, the tubes have a greater wall thickness towards the ends (for adequate strength and resistance to the heat when joining the tubes) than elsewhere along the length of the tube, as shown in Fig. 17.3. The use of such tubes, referred to as butted tubes, results in a lighter, more responsive and comfortable bike.

Given adequate strength and rigidity, the lighter bike is distinctly more enjoyable to ride, even if the difference seems minor relative to the total weight of bike and rider. This is due to the fact that, unlike the rider's own body weight, most of the weight of the bicycle (and any accessories and luggage you may be carrying) should be considered 'dead' weight or mass. Essentially, this is unsprung mass, which is not cushioned, as the equivalent weight of a car or motorcycle. Nor can it be transferred or shifted, as is the case for the rider's weight, which can be raised off the saddle in response to anticipated road shocks.

Another desirable feature, besides high strength and low weight, is adequate lateral and torsional rigidity of the bike. Rigidity means absence of flexibility. On a rigid bike, there is little deformation in response to a force applied to it at one point. Inadequate rigidity leads to the propagation of vibra-

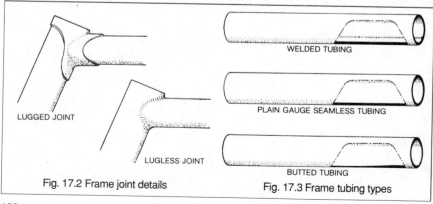

LUGGED JOINT

LUGLESS JOINT

WELDED TUBING

PLAIN GAUGE SEAMLESS TUBING

BUTTED TUBING

Fig. 17.2 Frame joint details   Fig. 17.3 Frame tubing types

tions, oscillations and swaying, particularly while riding fast on poor road surfaces or when changing direction abruptly. Unfortunately, rigidity is largely affected by some of the same factors as weight: for a given material and tube diameter, the rigidity decreases with decreasing wall thickness. As long as you use the bike only for unloaded cycling on normal roads, there'll be no problem of flexing, but it becomes critical when riding hard on poorly surfaced roads or with luggage, where slightly heavier frames are in order.

The most effective way to achieve greater rigidity is to increase the diameter of the tubes. Whereas a 20% increase in wall thickness only leads to a proportional 20% increase in rigidity, the effect of a 20% greater outside diameter, even with an unchanged wall thickness, is on the order of 70%. Both methods lead to the same 20% weight increase. This is the reason why the frame's down tube, which is most heavily subjected to torsional forces, is always made with a greater diameter than the other main tubes. It is also the reason most mountain bikes use bigger diameter frame tubes.

A third factor to keep in mind with regard to rigidity, is the material used for the tubes. On the one hand, all types of steel, from the cheapest and weakest to the strongest and most exotic, have the same inherent rigidity. Given the same diameter and wall thickness, the tubes are equally rigid, whatever kind of steel is used. On the other hand, aluminum with all its alloys is considerably less rigid. Consequently, an aluminum frame should have tubes that have a greater wall thickness (required to compensate for this material's lower strength anyway) as well as a greater outside diameter, if it is to be satisfactory.

The bicycle's frame geometry also affects its rigidity. The longer the individual tubes, the more flexible they become. This is the reason why racing frames, which use light tubes, are made as compact as they are.

Within certain limitations, the bicycle manufacturer is at liberty to select geometry, wall thickness and tube diameters to achieve the desired combination of strength, weight and rigidity required for a particular bike.

Only the diamond shaped frame gives the required rigidity. That applies to bikes for men and for women alike, and all special women's models (as well as tandems) without a horizontal top tube are potentially dangerous at higher speeds. Oddly enough, that applies particularly if the bike is made with high strength tubing, since it will have thinner walls.

Special frame designs and materials should be considered carefully. Moun-

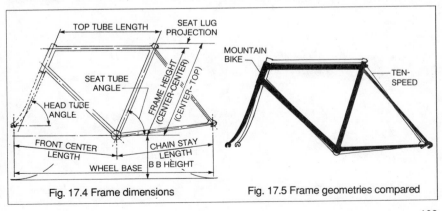

Fig. 17.4 Frame dimensions   Fig. 17.5 Frame geometries compared

tain bikes, quite suitable for many fitness uses, tend to have tubes of greater diameters, usually welded together without lugs. This makes them quite satisfactory, despite their generous dimensions. Aluminum frames must also have tubes of greater diameters, as well as a greater wall thickness. Since aluminum is so much lighter than steel, the overall weight will still be quite low.

Frame Dimensions

A bicycle's nominal size is determined by the frame size, which is defined as the length of the seat tube. Unfortunately, different manufacturers measure this dimension differently, as shown in Fig. B of Table 1 in the Appencix. In the English speaking world, the distance between the center of the bottom bracket and the top of the seat lug used to be quoted. It is becoming more customary to follow the French custom of measuring between the center of the bottom bracket and the center of the top tube. The same frame will be quoted as being 15mm, or about $^1/_2$ inch smaller in the latter case than in the former.

To select a frame of the right size, you can either use the advice contained in Table 1 in the Appendix, or you can try

out some frames for fit. With wheels of the correct size installed, the top tube should be at such a height that you can straddle it with both feet flat on the ground, wearing thin-soled shoes with minimal heels. Most people seem to buy a bike that is too big. When in doubt, I would suggest you deviate on the smaller, rather than on the larger side.

A mountain bike may have slightly more generous dimensions and clearances, including shallower angles between the horizontal and the seat tube and steering axis, as shown in Fig. 17.5, but with a shorter seat tube (resulting in a lower top tube).

The racing or fitness bike frame probably need not be equipped with many of the threaded bosses and lugs for the installation of accessories such as racks and fenders (in Britain called carriers and mud guards, respectively). However, you'll still want mounts for a water bottle and most of the other ones may prove useful someday.

The Steering System

This is the assembly of parts that keeps the bike on track and balanced, by allowing the rotational plane of the front wheel to pivot relative to the rest of the bike. As

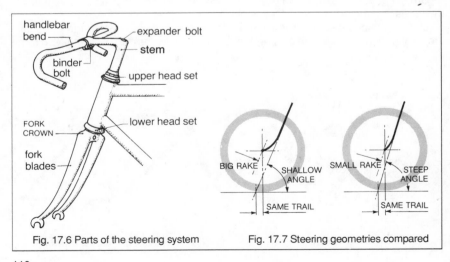

Fig. 17.6 Parts of the steering system   Fig. 17.7 Steering geometries compared

shown in Fig. 17.6, it comprises the fork, headset bearings, handlebar stem or extension, and the handlebars.

The Front Fork

The fork consists of two blades, terminating in fork- ends or front drop-outs, a fork crown and a steerer tube (or fork shaft), which is threaded at one end to accept the adjustable parts of the headset. The fork should be of similar materials to those used for a good. frame: strong alloy tubing, brazed onto the fork crown and with relatively thick fc ᶥk-ends.

Compared to a mountain bike or a touring machine, the racing or fitness bike should have less off-set, or rake. This is necessary to achieve the same steering characteristics, as shown in Fig 17.7. Typical values for a racing bike are a steerer tube angle of 73—74 degrees and a rake of 45—50mm.

If the steerer tube angle is smaller, which provides a more cushioned ride and is desirable on rough roads, the fork rake should be correspondingly greater to achieve the same steering characteristics.

In a collision, the fork will generally be the first thing to get damaged. Although such a bent fork can sometimes be straightened again, it will be smart to check with a bike mechanic, rather than experimenting around yourself. When in doubt, have a new fork installed.

The length of the fork's steerer tube is a function of the frame size. There are two distinct threading standards in use: French and English. The latter standard is used on most bikes. Nowadays, even some frames made for export by French manufacturers are originally supplied with English threading. It will be a good idea to take the old fork and a matching threaded part of the headset along when replacing a bent fork.

The Headset

The headset, shown in Fig. 17.8, consists of a double set of ball bearings. These are installed at the upper and lower ends of the head tube, with the matching parts fixed on the fork crown and screwed onto the threaded part of the steerer tube, respectively. The headset should be adjusted if the steering is either too loose or too tight. Proceed as follows:

1. Loosen the big locknut on the upper headset bearing by about 3—4 turns.
2. Unscrew the lock washer far enough to allow turning the bearing race immediately below.
3. Tighten or loosen the adjustable race as required, by turning it

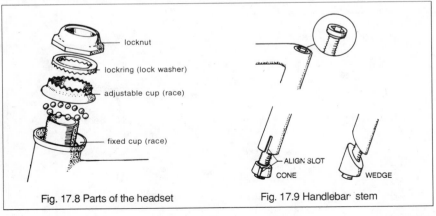

Fig. 17.8 Parts of the headset
locknut
lockring (lock washer)
adjustable cup (race)
fixed cup (race)
ALIGN SLOT
CONE
WEDGE
Fig. 17.9 Handlebar stem

clockwise or counterclockwise, respectively.

4. Put the lock washer in place and tighten the locknut, while holding the adjustable race.
5. If problems persist, see a bike shop.

Handlebars and Stem

The handlebars are attached to the fork's steerer tube by means of an L-shaped piece called handlebar stem. The lower end of this device fits inside the steerer tube. As shown in Fig. 17.9, a wedge or cone-shaped part can be pulled into the stem to clamp the two parts together by tightening the expander bolt. The latter is reached from the top and is generally operated by means of a hexagonal bar tool, referred to as allan key. At least 65mm (2.5 in) of the stem must remain contained inside the steerer tube for safety reasons.

The handlebar proper, also referred to as handlebar bend, is held in a split or otherwise clamped portion at the forward end of the stem. Here it is clamped by tightening a second bolt, referred to as binder bolt. Stems are generally made of aluminum alloy and are available in several different extension lengths. A different stem size may be necessary to adapt the distance between saddle and handlebars to the rider for maximum comfort, as was described in Chapter 2.

Handlebar bends are generally made of aluminum tubing. They are available in several distinct shapes, ranging from the wide flat things installed on mountain bikes to the narrow and deep models used on pure racing machines. For fitness bikes, some people prefer a model with a flat extension pointing forward, as used by some triathletes.

The middle part of the handlebars must be reinforced by an interior or exterior reinforcing sleeve (resulting in a section of greater diameter) over a length of at least 5cm (2 in) to eliminate the chance of breaking the bar at the point where it projects from the stem. Handlebar bend and stem must be matched, since handlebar diameters vary from one make and model to the other.

The drop bar is finished off by wrapping cloth or plastic handlebar tape around it. Alternately, you may choose to install flexible foam plastic sleeves. The latter solution appears to be most comfortable for cycling on less than perfect road surfaces. The open ends of the handlebar bend are closed off by inserting plastic plugs.

Saddle and Seat Post

Certainly if you are relatively new to cycling, the saddle or seat had better be comfortable. Most beginning cyclists

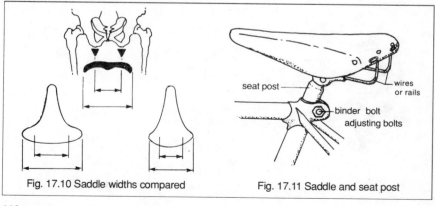

Fig. 17.10 Saddle widths compared   Fig. 17.11 Saddle and seat post

prefer to sit more upright than is customary for bicycle racing. This results in more weight resting on the saddle and more difficulty lifting the weight to relieve pain. Consequently, a different saddle design may be required. In general, a good touring or mountain bike saddle will do the trick. This should be somewhat wider in the back, though still as long and narrow in the front as the racing saddle. In particular women, who usually have a wider pelvis then most men, may need a wide, padded model. See

Fig. 17.10 for seat width details.

Fig. 17.11 shows the way the saddle is attached to the frame at the seat lug by means of a seat post, referred to as seat pin or seat pillar in Britain. The attachment bolts that hold the saddle to the seat post may be either on top, underneath or by the side of the seat clip that holds the saddle wires to the seat post.

The seat post should be of a model that allows fine adjustment of the position and the angle relative to the horizontal plane. Select one of the micro-adjustable models, as shown in Fig. 17.12. The seat post diameter should match the inside diameter of the seat tube, being 27.2mm on most quality frames built with butted tubing (except mountain bikes). The seat post is held at the right height by clamping the split seat lug around it when the seat binder bolt is tightened. The seat post should be so long that at least 65mm (2.5 in) is held inside the seat lug for safety reasons. See Chapter 2 for a step-by-step description of the saddle adjustment procedure.

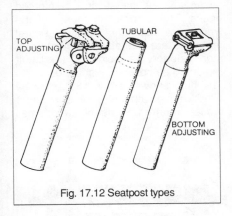

Fig. 17.12 Seatpost types

18. The Bicycle's Other Components

In the present chapter, the remaining components will be described in the same functional groups mentioned in Chapter 16: wheels, drivetrain, gearing system and brakes. Any accessories will be treated separately in Chapter 19. In addition, the gearing system, which is handled here summarily, was covered more fully in Chapter 4.

Some elementary maintenance instructions are included here for the components discussed. This is only done in those cases where it seems relevant in the context of a book like this. When you get into trouble *en route* because you have a flat (referred to as a puncture in Britain) or the chain comes off, you'll want to know what to do about it. On the other hand, there are numerous other possible maintenance or repair jobs that are not relevant here. You can get full information from my *Bicycle Repair Book*, while the less ambitious may choose to take their machine to a bike store.

The Wheels

A typical bicycle wheel is shown in Fig. 18.1. It is a spoked wheel with regular wired-on tires, which consist of a separate inner tube and a tire cover that is held tight in a deep bedded metal rim by means of metal-wire- reinforced beads. The other components of the wheel are hub and spokes. Wheel problems are perhaps the most common category of incidents, and their repair will be covered in some detail.

The hub, shown in Fig. 18.2, may be either a high flange or a low flange model (referred to as big and small

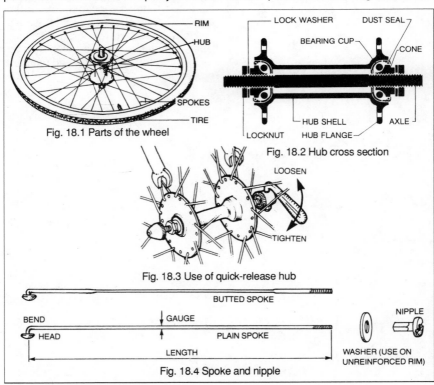

Fig. 18.1 Parts of the wheel

RIM
HUB
SPOKES
TIRE

Fig. 18.2 Hub cross section

LOCK WASHER   DUST SEAL
BEARING CUP
CONE
HUB SHELL   AXLE
LOCKNUT   HUB FLANGE

Fig. 18.3 Use of quick-release hub

LOOSEN
TIGHTEN

Fig. 18.4 Spoke and nipple

BUTTED SPOKE
BEND   GAUGE
HEAD   PLAIN SPOKE
LENGTH
NIPPLE
WASHER (USE ON UNREINFORCED RIM)

flange, respectively, in Britain). On most bikes the hubs have quick-release levers, allowing easy wheel removal (see Fig. 18.3).

The spokes, shown in Fig. 18.4, should be of stainless steel, and there are usually 36 of them per wheel. Each spoke is held to the rim by means of a screwed-on nipple, which should be kept tightened to maintain the spoke under tension, which actually prevents a lot of spoke breakages. The spokes run from the hub to the rim in one of several distinct patterns. Fig. 18.5 shows three-cross and four-cross spoking patterns.

The length of the spoke is measured as shown in the illustration Fig. 18.4 and depends on the wheel size, the type of hub, and the spoking pattern. The thickness is usually 1.8mm (or 15 gauge) on a sports or racing bike. Butted spokes have a thinner section in the middle and are as strong as regular spokes that are as thick as their thickest section (the lower gauge number in their size designation). If a spoke should break, get it replaced as soon as possible.

The Rims

For a sports bike of any quality, the rims must be of aluminum. In addition to the weight advantage, aluminum provides much better wet weather braking than chrome plated steel rims. Fig. 18.6 il-

lustrates the rim with a tire installed.

The spoke holes should be reinforced by means of ferrules. To protect the tube, a piece of tape should cover the part of the rim bed where the spoke nipples would otherwise touch the inner tube.

Wheel Truing

If the wheel is bent, proceed as follows to straighten it by retensioning certain spokes, as shown in Fig. 18.7:

1. Check just where it is off-set to the left, where to the right, by turning it slowly while watching at a fixed reference point, such as the brake shoes. Mark the relevant sections.
2. Tighten LH spokes in the area where the rim is off-set to the RH side in half-turn steps, while loosening the ones on the LH side — and vice versa.
3. Repeat steps 1 and 2 until the wheel is true enough not to rub on the brakes. This will get you by but, unless you are quite good at it, I suggest you get the job done properly by a bike mechanic as soon as possible.

Tires and Tubes

The size of the tire defines the nominal size of the wheel. Adult sports and racing bikes usually have either 27 in or 700mm tires of a rather narrow section.

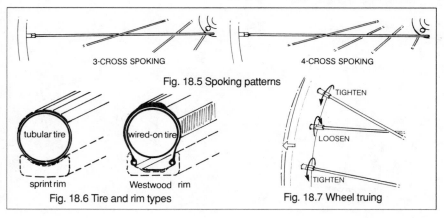

3-CROSS SPOKING   4-CROSS SPOKING

Fig. 18.5 Spoking patterns

tubular tire   wired-on tire

TIGHTEN

LOOSEN

TIGHTEN

sprint rim   Westwood rim

Fig. 18.6 Tire and rim types   Fig. 18.7 Wheel truing

The nominal sizes are a far cry from their actual dimensions: nominal 700mm tires normally measure anywhere from 666 to 686mm, depending on their width. Though these things are also known as 28 in tires, they are actually smaller than those of nominal size 27 in.

The inner tube should be of a size to match the tire. For any given size, it seems the lighter and thinner tube and tire give a better ride. Only in terrain with thorns and other frequent puncture causes, should the very thick thorn-proof tubes be used.

Tire and rim must match. The critical dimension determining tire interchangeability is the rim bed or rim shoulder dimension. For 27 in and 700mm tires this diameter should be 630mm and 622mm, respectively. Mountain bikes that roll on 26 in tires have rims of 559mm rim bed diameter, while hybrid bikes may have different sizes altogether.

As for the recommended tire width, it all depends on the terrain encountered. The minimum width suitable for normal use is probably 22mm, while 25 or even 28mm are good choices for use on mixed road surfaces. If you want to ride off-road or in regions where roads are maintained less scrupulously, hybrids and mountain bikes with tire widths anywhere from 35mm to 54mm are an excellent choice. Always look for a model with flexible sidewalls, which roll significantly lighter, especially on rough surfaces.

The tube is inflated by means of a valve, several types of which are illustrated in Fig. 18.8. By far the most suitable is the Presta valve, which requires much less force to inflate, though it can't be done by means of a gas station air hose. Unscrew the round nut at the tip before inflating, and tighten it again afterwards. Inflation pressure is the key to low rolling resistance and immunity to puncturing. Maintain at least the pressure quoted on the tire side wall, and don't hesitate to inflate at least the rear wheel by about 15% more than that minimum value.

Sooner or later, every cyclist gets a flat. It helps if you are able to handle this repair yourself. Carry a puncture kit, three tire irons (called tyre levers in Britain), a pump and perhaps a spare tube. The adhesive quality of the patches in your kit deteriorates over time, so I suggest replacing them once a year. Proceed as follows:

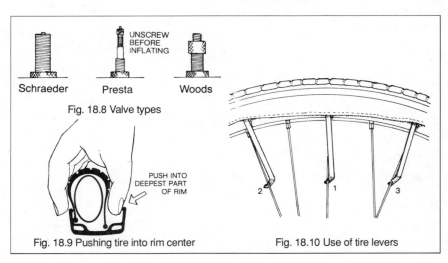

UNSCREW BEFORE INFLATING

Schraeder   Presta   Woods

Fig. 18.8 Valve types

PUSH INTO DEEPEST PART OF RIM

Fig. 18.9 Pushing tire into rim center

Fig. 18.10 Use of tire levers

Fixing a Flat

1. Remove the wheel from the bike. On a rear wheel, first select the gear with the small chainwheel and sprocket, then hold the chain with the derailleur back.

2. Check whether the cause is visible from the outside. In that case, remove it and mark its location, so you know where to work.

3. Remove the valve cap and lock-nut, unscrew the round nut (if you have a Presta valve).

4. Push the valve body in and work one side of the tire into the deeper center of the rim, as shown in Fig. 18.9.

5. Put a tire iron under the bead on that side, at some distance from the valve, then use it to lift the bead over the rim edge and hook it on a spoke, as shown in Fig. 18.10.

6. Do the same with the second tire iron two spokes to the left and with the third one two spokes over to the right. Now the first one will come loose, so you may use it in a fourth location, if necessary.

7. When enough of the tire sidewall is lifted over the rim, you can lift the rest over by hand.

8. Remove the tube, saving the valve until last, when it must be pushed back through the valve hole.

9. Try inflating and check where air escapes. If the hole is very small, so it can't be easily detected, pass the tube slowly past your eye, which is quite sensitive. If still no luck, dip the tube under water, a section at a time: the hole is wherever bubbles escape. Mark its location and dry the tire if appropriate. There may be more than just one hole.

10. Make sure the area around the patch is dry and clean, then roughen it with the sand paper or the scraper from the puncture kit and remove the resulting dust.

Treat an area slightly larger than the patch you want to use.

11. Quickly and evenly, spread a thin film of rubber solution on the treated area. Let dry about 3 minutes.

12. Remove the foil backing from the patch, without touching the adhesive side. Place it with the adhesive side down on the treated area, centered on the hole. Apply pressure over the entire patch to improve adhesion.

13. Sprinkle talcum powder from the patch kit over the treated area.

14. Inflate the tube and wait long enough to make sure the repair is carried out properly.

15. Meanwhile, check the inside of the tire and remove any sharp objects that may have caused the puncture. Also make sure no spoke ends project from the rim bed — file flush if necessary and cover with rim tape.

16. Let enough air out of the tube to make it limp but not completely empty. Then reinsert it under the tire, starting at the valve.

17. *With your bare hands*, pull the tire back over the edge of the rim, starting opposite the valve, which must be done last of all. If it seems too tight, work the part already installed deeper into the center of the rim bed, working around towards the valve from both sides.

18. Make sure the tube is not pinched between rim and tire bead anywhere, working and kneading the tire until the tube is free.

19. Install the valve locknut and inflate the tube to about a third its final pressure.

20. Center the tire relative to the rim, making sure it lies evenly all around on both sides.

21. Inflate to its final pressure, then install the wheel. If the tire is wider than the rim, you may have to

release the brake (just make sure you tighten it again afterwards). On the rear wheel, refer to point 1 above.

Note: If the valve leaks, or if the tube is seriously damaged, the entire tube must be replaced, which is done following the relevant steps of these same instructions. Replacement of the tire cover is done similarly.

The Drivetrain

The bicycle's drivetrain comprises the parts that transmit the power from the rider's legs to the rear wheel. The gearing system is often considered part of the drivetrain as well, but I have chosen to treat it separately.

The heart of the drivetrain is the crankset, referred to as chainset in Britain, which is installed in the frame's bottom bracket. It turns around a spindle or axle that is supported in ball bearings. The two types of bottom bracket bearing systems used on quality bicycles are the adjustable cup-and-cone type and the non-adjustable cartridge type, usually referred to as sealed bearing unit. These two varieties are depicted in Fig. 18.11 and Fig. 18.12, respectively.

On virtually all quality bikes built nowadays, the spindle has tapered square ends, matching correspondingly shaped recesses in the cranks. The cranks are held on the spindle by means of a bolt, covered by a dust cap in the crank. This method of attachment is referred to as cotterless and is shown in Fig. 18.13. Spindle lengths, bottom bracket widths, screw threading and taper shape all may differ, even if (different) models of the same make are installed. Consequently, all parts of the bottom bracket can only be replaced when the original and the matching parts are taken along to the shop, to make sure they fit as a system.

On a new bike, the cranks tend to come loose after some use, as they may at more infrequent intervals later on. For this reason, and for other maintenance or replacement work, I suggest you obtain a matching crank tool for the particular make and model installed on your bike. Check and tighten the cranks every 25 miles during the first 100 miles, and perhaps once a month afterwards.

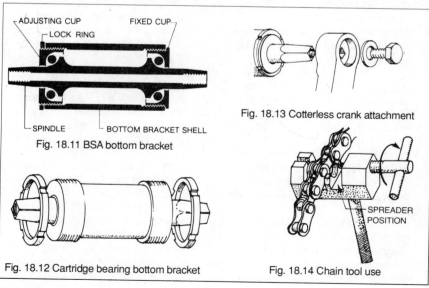

Fig. 18.11 BSA bottom bracket

Fig. 18.12 Cartridge bearing bottom bracket

Fig. 18.13 Cotterless crank attachment

Fig. 18.14 Chain tool use

Tighten Cotterless Crank

1. Remove the dust cap with any fitting tool (on most models a coin may be used).
2. Using the wrench part of the special crank tool, tighten the recessed bolt firmly, countering at the crank.
3. Reinstall the dust cap.

The cranks are generally made of aluminum and are available in several different lengths. Unless you have particularly long or short legs, the standard size of 17cm (about 7 in) will be quite satisfactory.

Chainrings

The RH crank has an attachment spider for installation of the chainrings, also called chainwheels. Racing and sports bikes usually have two, while mountain bikes have three chainrings. Check the attachment bolts of the chainrings from time to time, and tighten them evenly if necessary.

Most sports bikes and mountain bikes are equipped with non-round chainrings, such as the popular Shimano Biopace. They are claimed to help inex-perienced riders pedal more efficiently but have no advantage to anyone who has learned to pedal fast.

The Chain

The chain connects the crankset with the rear wheel, where a freewheel block with several different size sprockets is installed. The chain is routed as explained below. It must have the right length: it should neither hang loose nor tighten up excessively when using either of the extreme gearing combinations (big chainring with the biggest sprocket or small chainring with the smallest sprocket).

On derailleur bikes, an endless chain is used, which may be parted by removing one of the pins connecting two links. The same method is used to add or remove links to adjust the chain's length. It may be necessary to remove the chain for cleaning and lubrication. To do that, you will need a chain tool, which is used as illustrated in Fig. 18.14 and described below:

Chain Removal and Installation

1. Put the chain on a combination of a small chainwheel with a small

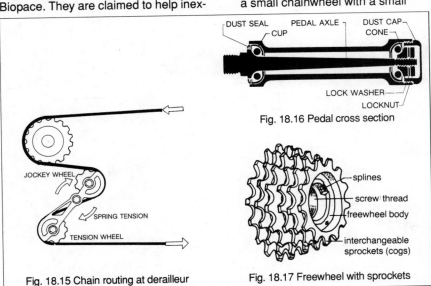

Fig. 18.15 Chain routing at derailleur

Fig. 18.16 Pedal cross section

Fig. 18.17 Freewheel with sprockets

sprocket, to release its tension.

2. Place the tool on one of the pins connecting two links, and turn it in by 6 turns.

3. Turn the handle of the tool back out and remove the tool from the chain.

4. Wriggle the chain apart.

5. Reinstall the chain, routing it around the derailleur per Fig. 18.15.

The Pedals

The pedals are installed at the ends of the cranks. Fig. 18.16 shows the guts of one. The threaded end is screwed in — the LH one with LH-thread, the RH one with normal RH-thread Either toeclips are used to hold the feet to the pedals, or a special clipless pedal with matching shoe.

The Freewheel

Depending on the make and type of rear wheel hub, the freewheel is either screwed on, or it is a separate unit integrated in the (special) hub, referred to as cassette type. Although the latter, of which the Shimano Cassette Freehub is the best know, are quite satisfactory in

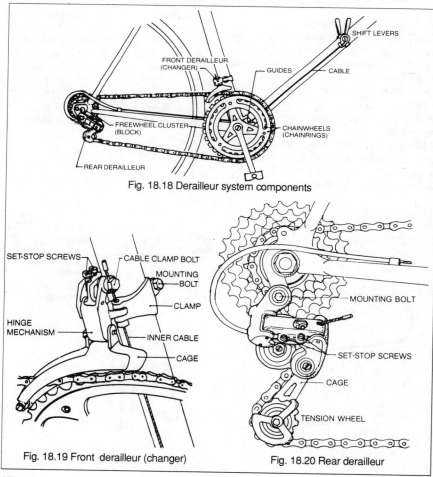

Fig. 18.18 Derailleur system components

Fig. 18.19 Front derailleur (changer)

Fig. 18.20 Rear derailleur

use, their disadvantage is that the entire wheel has to be replaced (or at least rebuilt) if the freewheel mechanism fails. Fig. 18.17 shows a common screwed-on freewheel with its sprockets, or cogs.

The Gearing System

In this section we'll discuss only the hardware, while the niceties of the system, including selection and handling, were described in Chapter 4.

A typical derailleur system is shown in Fig. 18.18. It consists of a front changer and a rear derailleur, which are operated by means of shift levers. The shifters may be installed either on the down tube, at the handlebar ends or, in the case of a bike with flat handlebars, on top of the bars. Other shift lever positions, such as at the stem, are inherently unsuitable, since they are not easily accessible without interfering with bike

handling. The shifters are connected to the changers by means of flexible cables that run over guides and, in the case of handlebar-mounted shifters, partly inside flexible outer cables.

The Derailleurs

The front changer or derailleur, shown in Fig. 18.19, is installed on the seat tube, either by means of a clip around the tube or by means of brazed-on lug. The rear derailleur, depicted in Fig. 18.20, is installed on the RH drop-out, which should have a threaded eye for this purpose, though adaptor plates are provided with most derailleurs to allow installing them on a bike without it. The chain is routed around the rear derailleur as shown in Fig. 18.15, while it simply runs through the changer's cage in the front.

The derailleurs shift the chain over sideways to engage a smaller or bigger

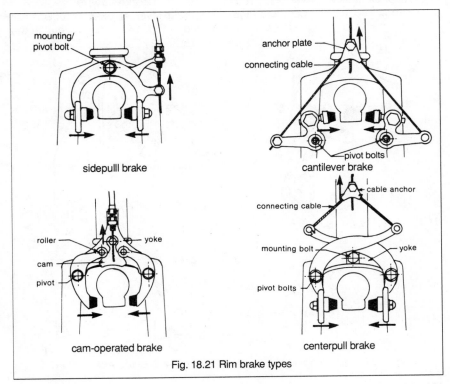

sidepulll brake

cantilever brake

cam-operated brake

centerpull brake

Fig. 18.21 Rim brake types

chainring or sprocket, while you continue to pedal forward with reduced pedal force. The combination of a large chainring and a small sprocket provides a high gear, suitable for easy terrain conditions. Engaging a small chainring and a large sprocket provides a low gear, required for going up an incline, starting off or riding against a head wind. See Chapter 4 for further details.

The Brakes

There are four different types of rim brakes in use for sports bikes. Fig. 18.21 shows the various types, which may be referred to as centerpull, sidepull, cantilever, and cam-operated brakes, respectively.

On the sidepull brake, the brake arms pivot around the attachment bolt, while they pivot around separate bosses installed on a common yoke on the centerpull brake. On the cantilever brake and the frame-mounted cam-operated brake, the pivots are installed on bosses

that are attached directly to the fork or seat stays.

The force applied by pulling the lever is transmitted to the brake unit by means of flexible cables. These cables are partly contained in flexible outer cables and restrained at anchor points on the frame. The force is transmitted to the parts of the brake unit to which the cable is attached. A pivoting action then pulls the ends of the brake arms with the brake blocks against the sides of the rim to create the drag that slows down the bike.

On most sports and racing bikes, sidepull brakes are installed, while cantilevers and cam-operated brakes, as well as a particular variant of the centerpull brake, called U-brake, are used on mountain bikes, hybrids and touring bikes.

Brake Levers

The brake lever, an example of which is shown in Fig. 18.22, should match the

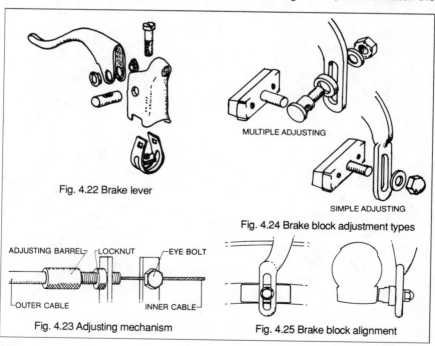

Fig. 4.22 Brake lever

MULTIPLE ADJUSTING

SIMPLE ADJUSTING

Fig. 4.24 Brake block adjustment types

ADJUSTING BARREL LOCKNUT   EYE BOLT

OUTER CABLE   INNER CABLE

Fig. 4.23 Adjusting mechanism

Fig. 4.25 Brake block alignment

handlebar type used and it should be easy to reach, while allowing full application of the brake. The type of lever designed for mountain bikes is quite suitable for any bike with flat handlebars, providing the attachment clamp matches the bar diameter. For drop handlebars, models with extension levers are not satisfactory, even for beginners, since they are insufficiently rigid and often shorten the regular handle's range of travel.

Brake Blocks

The brake blocks should preferably be of a composition material that provides adequate braking even in the rain, which is just not the case with any kind of plain rubber brake blocks. Contrary to popular belief, longer brake blocks are not better but poorer than shorter ones, given the same material. Depending on the type of brake used, the brake blocks may be installed in one of the two basic types of brake shoes illustrated in Fig. 18.24, which are adjustable in one and two planes, respectively.

Brake Test

To make sure the brakes work properly, try them out separately at walking speed, which is perfectly safe and still gives a representative test of the deceleration reached with each brake. Used alone while riding the bike, the rear brake must be strong enough to skid the wheel when applied firmly. The front brake should decelerate the bike so much that the rider notices the rear wheel lifting off when it is applied fully. If their performance is inadequate, carry out the adjustment described in the next section.

Brake Adjustment

We will assume the brake must be adjusted because its performance is insufficient. In this case, the cable tension must be increased by decreasing its length. Should the brake touch the rim even when not engaged, the opposite must be done to lengthen the cable slightly. The adjuster mechanism is shown in Fig. 18.23.

Before starting, check to make sure the brake blocks lie on the rim properly over their entire width and length when the brake is applied, as shown in Fig. 18.25. Ideally, the front of the brake block should touch the rim just a little earlier than the back. If necessary, adjust by loosening the brake block bolt, moving the block as appropriate. Retighten it while holding the brake block in the right position. If necessary, the brake block may be replaced, after which it must be adjusted as well.

Adjusting procedure
1. Release brake quick-release.
2. Loosen locknut on the adjusting mechanism.
3. While holding the locknut, screw the barrel adjuster out by several turns; then tighten the quick-release again.
4. Check the brake tension: the brake must grab the rim firmly when a minimum of 2cm ($^3/_4$ in) clearance remains between the brake handle and the handlebars.
5. If necessary, repeat steps 1—4 until the brake works properly.
6. Tighten the locknut again, while holding the adjusting barrel to stop it from turning.

19. Other Equipment

In this chapter, we shall examine the accessories that can be installed on the bike and the various other items that may be handy in your fitness program. Much of the bicycle equipment described here is intended for specific uses and not necessarily recommended for use by every cyclist all the time. Just the same, it will benefit all riders to know what is available and how to select the right accessories either now or later.

In addition to the more general bicycle accessories described in the sections that follow, there are a few items particularly helpful in any fitness program. These will be briefly introduced first.

Bicycle Computer

This is the rather immodest name generally used for an electronic speedometer. Generally consisting of a readout unit to be mounted on the handlebars and a sensor that picks up the impulses from a magnet installed on the front wheel, this is your basic guide to riding speed. Get one with as few buttons as possible and remove it off the bike whenever you have to leave it unguarded for any time.

More sophisticated versions have (or can be expanded with) special features that measure the pedaling rate and sometimes even your pulse or heart rate. Each supplementary function requires additional sensors and wires. For conscious training they can be very helpful though, since the heartrate is the guide to effective training.

Pulse Rate Monitor

This is a handy gadget disguised as a wrist watch that tells you what your heart is doing without having additional wires running around the bike. Battery powered and light to carry, this is handier than any other method of keeping track of your performance. If you're not into gadgets, you can choose to count

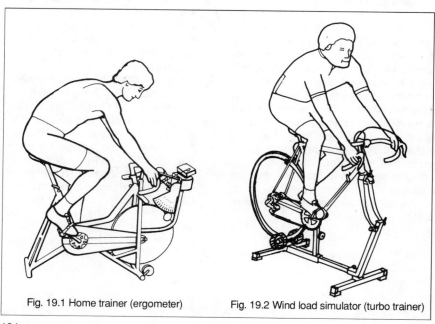

Fig. 19.1 Home trainer (ergometer)   Fig. 19.2 Wind load simulator (turbo trainer)

out the heart rate following the method described in Chapter 1.

Home Trainer

Illustrated in Fig. 19.1, this is the old-fashioned and in my opinion not very satisfactory device to allow indoor bike training. It's a crude stationary device with a bicycle seat and handlebars and a big flywheel with a variable mechanical or electrical resistance to vary the load, and a panel that shows how fast you are going or how much effort you are putting in. These things are still available, but I suggest instead using the wind load simulator described below.

Wind Load Simulator

Shown in Fig. 19.2 and also known as turbo-trainer, this device does the same job, but better. It is a stand with a clamp to hold your own bike. The bike's rear wheel drives a set of wind turbines or a electro-magnetic resistane. The advantages include the better position and ergonomic conditions provided by the use of your own familiar bike and the fact that the resistance provided by the wind turbines is more similar to the speed-dependent resistance when riding the bike

The mostmodern of these items are referred to as cyclo-computers actually include a computer-controlled variable resistance, which can be programmed to simulate any kind of ride, including hills, headwinds and the like. Even if you settle for a model without computer, I suggest you obtain one with an integratedi output indicator, showing how hard you are working at any time. In combination with your pulse monitor this is as good as having your own physiology lab. Ideal, not only for off-season indoor training, but also for monitoring your performance and progress.

Weight and Muscle Training Equipment

Cycling is a weird sort of movement. Un-like running, swimming or rowing, it loads only one of the muscles in each matched pair, and starves some muscles altogether for variable-length work. The result is that these muscles get inadequate development, or at a minimum that your legs feel like pudding after a long, hard ride.

As we shall see in the chapter devoted to muscle work, there is a real need to develop some of the muscles that are used only isometrically in cycling. This can be done by conscious calisthenics and other gymnastic exercises. However, it can also be done by using weight training methods. A pair of dumbells and a few other simple devices can come in useful for this purpose.

Another simple device, not commercially available but easily made, is the slant board, shown in Fig. 19.3. Stand on it toes up, heels down for a period of 10 to 20 minutes a day, especially on heavy riding days, while doing something else, and your muscles and joints will be much better balanced. Some advice on weight and muscle training and other methods of muscle training are included in the training chapters of Part II.

Other Accessories

The following descriptions deal with all those accessories that make the bike suitable for year-round biking, which is the key to fitness. They may be readily installed on the bike when purchased, or installed at a later date.

In order to install accessories on a bicycle without such special provisions, you will have to rely on provisional clamps and the like. It will be advisable to attach any such clamps only after installing a rubber patch from the bicycle tire patch kit around the bike's tubing locally. This not only protects paintwork or metal finish, it also prevents the clamp from slipping or twisting. Do not use self-adhesive tape for this purpose, since it will slip over time, whereas a tire patch, applied just like you would do to fix a flat tire, will stay in place firmly.

By way of maintenance of most accessories, you merely have to make sure the things are not broken or loose. Tighten the various attachment bolts from time to time, preferably on a regular basis. To make sure bolts do not come loose, I suggest you use washers and locknuts wherever possible.

Bags and Racks

For longer trips, certainly once cycling has become more to you than just a method to keep fit, you may want to carry luggage. And that is best done with the use of racks or carriers, though some bags are available that attach directly to the bike. Either way is preferable to carrying things in a backpack, which hinders you while cycling.

Luggage racks are available for the front and the rear. Generally, the rear rack allows carrying relatively large bags by the side and on top, while the one in the front is smaller, being attached to the fork. Interesting only when you go on longer tours.

Whatever their type, make sure the racks can be attached very firmly to the bike. Preferably, brazed-on attachment lugs or bosses should be installed on the bike, exactly matching the dimensions of the particular rack used. That may become a bit of a problem when replacing the rack on a used bike or when installing a rack on a bike for the first time. However, a certain degree of standardization has taken place. Most manufacturers design their equipment in line with the attachment details of the racks produced by Jim Blackburn.

Fenders

Although many cyclists in America abhor the idea of installing fenders, or mud guards, on their bicycle, I suggest you use them in rainy areas or rainy seasons. Even if it isn't raining while you ride, the spray from a wet road is just as irritating. You may not want to bother if you live in a region where it simply doesn't ever rain for a period of several months. Even then, you would be well advised to get fenders, though you may hold off on installing them until the rainy season starts. Cycling in the rain or on

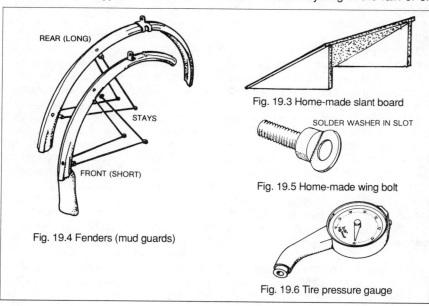

REAR (LONG)

STAYS

FRONT (SHORT)

Fig. 19.4 Fenders (mud guards)

Fig. 19.3 Home-made slant board

SOLDER WASHER IN SLOT

Fig. 19.5 Home-made wing bolt

Fig. 19.6 Tire pressure gauge

wet roads after it has rained is not as bad as some people think, and it will certainly be less miserable when you are equipped for it.

Yes, you can ride in the rain, or on a wet road after the rain, on a bike without fenders. But you'll be dead miserable. A spray of muddy water will stain your back and your bike; another jet of water will be shooting at your feet, and there's no way to get comfortable that way. Though you may still need rain gear to keep the rain off the top, you'll find fenders at least keep you reasonably dry and clean from below.

Fig. 19.4 shows typical fenders. At the top, they are attached to the brake bolt behind the front fork and in front of the bridge connecting the seat stays, for front and rear fenders, respectively. In the rear, a second point of attachment is by means of a clip over the bridge just behind the bottom bracket. Finally, they are held by means of rather thin rods, called stays, to the front fork-ends and rear drop-outs, respectively.

Install plain washers between bolts or nuts and the various clips or stays. The fender should be mounted in such a way that about 2cm ($^3/_4$ in) radial and at least 1cm ($^3/_8$ in) lateral clearance remains between the tires on the one hand and the fender with its stays on the other. If the fender is either crooked, too close, or too far from the wheel, do not adjust it by bending the stays. Instead, undo the clamping point and move the stays in or out to suit, after which the bolt is tightened again. Any excessive protrusions should be cut off first.

If you choose to install fenders only occasionally, removable attachments are easy enough to make, as shown in Fig. 19.5. If the bike has caliper brakes, attached by means of single bolts in fork crown and rear brake bridge, replace their attachment nuts by two thinner nuts, between which the fender clip is clamped. Install and tighten both nuts, even when the fender is not installed,

since a single thin nut is not adequate to restrain the brake.

Fenders may be either of plastic or of metal. The lightest satisfactory fenders available are the plastic models made by Bluemels (now part of a company called SKS).

To really keep the water that is splashed up from the road at the front wheel from your feet, you will need a mud flap installed at the bottom of the front fender. Very few models available in the US have one of these things attached, but you can make your own, using a 15—20cm (6—8 in) square piece of flexible, but relatively thick plastic sheet.

Lights

Next to fenders, bicycle lights are perhaps the most maligned accessories in the US. In many other countries they are obligatory — for good reasons, as you will appreciate If you have ever experienced how an unlit cyclist appears out of nowhere in your car headlights or when riding your bike during darkness or at dusk, you will perhaps appreciate just how dangerous it can be to go without. The fact that you didn't run into the turkey does not prove that it is safe to go without lights: the risk is infinitely greater without than it is with lights.

Many cyclists argue they never ride in the dark anyway. However, from experience I can report that just about every one who told me that was not only lying, he was also playing with his life. Sooner or later, you will want to leave the place you are staying without being able to return before dark. Or your day's trip will take you longer than expected. In short, though you may not plan on using lights, you should have them available in case you do need them.

Bicycle lights may be either battery operated or powered by means of a generator, referred to as a dynamo in Britain. Generator operated models are almost invariably installed permanently, while most battery models may be simply removed from the bike. The removability may be good or bad: bad if it's stolen when you do leave it on, good if you can avoid somebody messing around with it by taking it off yourself. Even if the lights are not stolen or vandalized, they may get damaged, so it will be wise to check their operation regularly and to tighten all mechanical and electric connections.

It is possible to use an easily removable form of dynamo lighting. In that case, you will have to make do without a rear light, which is perhaps justified if you use a really big reflector in the rear and make sure it is never obstructed. Removable units are installed to the front fork and consist of a dynamo with light attached.

The many possible trouble sources of most generator lighting systems and the physical resistance caused by their mechanical inefficiency are the reasons why many cyclists prefer battery lights. The batteries and the bulbs must match the light unit: some use a single flat (and hard-to-get) European 4.5 volt battery, other models two D-cells, still others two C-cells. Special lights, powered by a large rechargeable battery, are also available. In general, the larger the battery, the more powerful and longer lasting the light is likely to be.

Normal carbon-zinc batteries produce a gradually decreasing electric output over the battery's life. Replace such batteries when the light begins to dim — don't wait until the thing is virtually dead. Rechargeable NiCad (nickel-cadmium) batteries stay equally bright much longer, to go out quite suddenly when the charge is depleted. So make sure the battery is charged regularly, or that you have a charged spare with you, since there is no warning when the light will go off. If you have to leave the bike out in the rain, you'd better remove the batteries and store them in a dry place. This stops them from swelling up, becoming useless themselves and damaging the light unit to boot.

Make sure to get correctly rated bulbs for the batteries used, both in terms of voltage and wattage or amperage. I suggest using the krypton or halogen gas filled bulbs, the latter are brighter when new, while both types stay equally bright throughout their useful lifespan, whereas regular bulbs dim to less than half their original and rated light output.

Reflectors

In addition to lights, some reflectors are quite useful. But they can not completely replace lights, and some reflectors are of no protective benefit whatsoever. The CPSC requirement that all bicycles sold in the US must be equipped with a whole plethora of reflectors is a big step in the wrong direction, promptly followed by equally inept agencies in other countries. It gives people the false conviction to be adequately protected with the wrong equipment. Add to that the particular models prescribed show up brightly under certain obvious but irrelevant conditions, and you've been fooled. Useful is only a big rear reflector, even as a substitute for a rear light. It must be mounted where it can not be obstructed.

Pump and Tire Gauge

You will need to keep your tires inflated properly. Don't count on having gas stations handily available to inflate your tires, and don't just guess at the pressure. For efficient and trouble-free cycling, an adequate tire pressure is important, both to minimize rolling resistance and to protect the tire against damage. If you are experienced enough to have developed a calibrated thumb, you may do without a tire pressure gauge, shown in Fig. 19.6, to check the pressure, but nobody should go without a pump.

The pump should be a model suitable for developing an adequately high pressure. Depending on tire size and design, that may be anywhere from 3—7 bar (45—105 psi) gauge pressure. Be guided by the pressure quoted on the tire sidewalls as an absolute minimum and don't hesitate to inflate the one in the rear up to 15 psi more for use on normal roads.

In the preceding chapter, I recommended getting tires with Presta valves (also referred to as French valves). Make sure both the pump and the gauge have a connection that corresponds to the type of valve used. Don't use a pump with a flexible hose connector, since the air trapped in the hose makes it impossible to reach an adequate pressure with a normal hand pump. For quick tire inflation at home you may keep a big stand pump, which has enough volume to work fine with a flexible hose connector.

Nowadays, pumps are mostly designed to clamp directly between the bike's top tube and bottom bracket along the seat tube. These are referred to as frame-fit pumps, and are available in several sizes to match a range of frame sizes each. Many bikes have a peg along the bottom of the top tube — there the pump fits between it and the seat lug.

If the pump does not work properly, tighten the screwed nozzle and if necessary replace the underlying rubber washer that seals around the valve, taking care to install it the right way round, so it doesn't leak even more afterwards.

Off course, pumping up a tire is work, and America would not be America if the CO_2 cartridge inflator had not been developed for bicycle tire inflation. And of course many fitness-seekers are so busy upgrading their physique that they can't find the time and the energy to pump up their tires by hand. If you insist, go ahead, just allow me to state it's ridiculous.

Water Bottle and Cage

Here's another useful accessory, especially in hot weather and for longer rides.

Fig. 19.7 shows both a bottle and the cage in which it is installed on the bike. In case your bike lacks the bosses, most bottle cages are sold complete with a pair of rather crude clips to put around a frame tube. If you need to mount the thing that way, first stick a tire patch around the frame tube, as explained before.

Bike water bottles are available in cheap and fancy versions and in small and large sizes. The more expensive bottles should have the kind of spout illustrated, which is operated by pulling the central part out and closed off by pushing it back in. Don't drink by sucking at the spout: instead, hold the bottle inclined with the spout down at one or two inches from the open mouth and squirt the water in by squeezing on the bottle.

There are some interesting bottle variants on the market these days. One of these actually squirts when held upright, due to an internal tube that runs from the spout to the bottom of the bottle. Then there are thermos bottles, insulated with a foam material, and extra large bottles. One way to keep a cold drink of water cool is by wrapping a cloth (such as a sock) around it. Moisten this cloth occasionally by squirting some water out, so that evaporation will draw enough heat out of the bottle to keep the contents cool. Of course, that is only practical with water. You may also want a bottle with a more nourishing liquid, such as fruit juice. In winter, I use the insulated thermos bottle and keep a hot liquid in it.

The Lock

Unfortunately, a good lock is an essential accessory for any kind of cycling, except for trips that are so short that you know you can walk the bike back if you run into a problem. The very best lock is barely good enough to hold on to your bike in many parts of the world nowadays. The best locks are the large U-locks, such as the ones made by Kryptonite and Citadel. They may be installed by means of a special bracket.

Don't just lock the bike onto itself, but secure it to some immovable object. Though the U-locks fit nicely around many street furnishings, you may also want to use a strong cable or chain with end loops or shackles big enough to fit the lock. This allows you to tie the bike up to something bigger. Make sure to select an object from which the lock can not be lifted off: a chain around a parking meter is of little use if the cable can be slipped over the top.

Even with the best lock, you may not be able to completely protect your bike, equipment and accessories against vandalism and theft of individual items. The smartest thing to do is to be totally paranoid and suspect thieves and thugs everywhere and anytime. Never go anywhere without securing your gear. If at all possible, don't leave your equipment out of sight. When riding in a group, you may decide to take turns keeping an eye on things. At least keep the most valuable items in a bag that you always take with you on your body.

Warning Devices
When travelling on a narrow, winding mountain road, you may want to alert others to your presence for your own protection. You can use a compressed gas powered sound horn that can be carried in your back pocket. If you cycle on paths frequented by pedestrians, runners, roller skaters, dog walkers and casual cyclists, you may prefer to use a bell or just rely on your voice, since it is less offensive, yet adequately audible

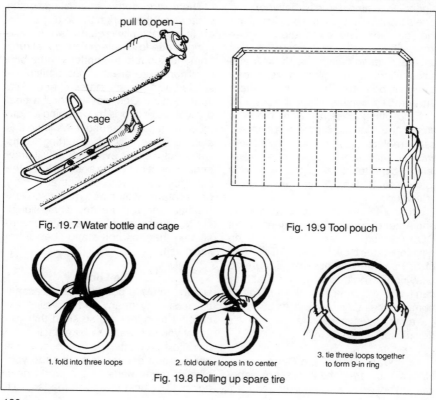

Fig. 19.7 Water bottle and cage

pull to open

cage

Fig. 19.9 Tool pouch

1. fold into three loops

2. fold outer loops in to center

3. tie three loops together to form 9-in ring

Fig. 19.8 Rolling up spare tire

under these circumstances.

Tools and Spares

Depending on a number of factors, you should carry some tools and spare parts on longer rides. How many you need depends on several factors, including the distance and the difficulty of the terrain, as well as the population and bike density of the region. In an area with plenty of gas stations and a bike shop every twenty miles, you do not need as many items as you should carry when crossing the desert. Here's a list of the essentials that should probably always be taken along on any longer trip away from home:

- A set of three tire levers;
- A tire patch kit, containing patches, rubber solution, chalk, sand paper, talcum powder and a piece of canvas to mend a damaged tire casing.;
- A small screw driver with a 4mm (^{3}/16 in) wide blade;
- A crescent wrench (adjustable spanner), 6 or 8 inches long;
- Allan keys in whatever sizes correspond to the recessed hexagon bolts used on your bike;
- A crank extractor tool, especially the wrench part, which will be needed to tighten a loose crank;
- A tube of waterless hand cleaner
- Cleaning rags to wipe your hands as well as protect or clean any messy parts before working on them.

Additionally, you may want to take the following special items on long trips:

- Spoke wrench (nipple spanner) to straighten a bent wheel;
- Chain rivet tool to take the chain apart and join it up again;
- A pair of small pliers, e.g. needle nose pliers with sharp cutters;
- Spare parts: spokes of correct length, brake cable, tube, chain links and lighting parts. If you also take a spare tire, turn it into three loops, as shown in Fig. 19.8.

When buying tools, consider that under the primitive roadside repair conditions, you should have the best tools available. Get quality tools. That means generally expensive tools, exactly fitting the parts in question. Don't let terms like 'economy tools' fool you: in the long run the best tools are more economical than any cheap tool will ever be, since the former lasts forever, while the latter quickly wears out and may actually damage the bike's components.

Tool Pouch

I suggest you carry the tools and spares in a pouch that holds all the tools you ever plan to carry and a few spare slots. If you can't buy one ready-made, it will be easy enough to sew your own. Be guided by Fig. 19.9, using a strong material such as denim. Allow enough space between the various items to enable you to roll it all together when it is full. On shorter trips, you may leave certain slots empty, to be used only for tools needed on longer trips, when the chances of needing them are greater.

20. Bicycle Clothing

In the present chapter, not only the cute, fashionable, colorful, tight-fitting bicycle clothing will be described, but also the kind of gear to wear when the weather is less than perfect. The same approach will be used in the next chapter, dealing with accessories.

Too many people limit their riding to periods with fair weather. Yes, it's more fun when the weather is nice. But you won't achieve much if you abandon the project whenever the sun goes in hiding. Get the clothing and equipment to also ride when the weather is less than perfect if you take it seriously. Surprisingly to some, it's even fun to ride in imperfect weather — less fun than it is when the sun shines, perhaps, but still a lot better than sitting at home waiting for the sun to come out.

Racing Dress

First we shall look at normal cycling wear. Bicycle clothing is probably the most functional gear ever designed for any sport, and though there'll be no need to ride around looking to all the world like Greg LeMond or Rebecca Twigg, it makes sense to aim at the same comfort that has been developed to accommodate racers. Besides, in recent years bicycle clothing — and fit-

ness clothing in general — has become high fashion in some circles. It has been developed thanks to the use of modern fabrics and bright colors to look good, rather than weird, as it did only a decade ago.

This gear has been designed the way it is to provide the freedom of movement, the control of temperature and humidity and the protection against chafing that allows a racer to continue non-stop for seven hours, covering 150 miles or more. That, I'm sure, will also be comfortable when riding half the distance at a lower speed.

I shall highlight the points that make the various items of bicycle clothing so suitable for their purpose. These will also be the things to watch out for when buying clothing that is not specifically designed for the purpose, to determine whether it will serve you anyway. You may refer to Fig. 20.1 for an idea of what a typical racing outfit looks like.

Shoes and Socks

The shoes are perhaps the single most important item that can make the difference between effective cycling and plodding along. Special bicycling shoes consist of light leather uppers with a thin but very stiff sole, generally with a metal

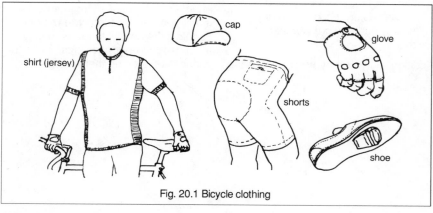

Fig. 20.1 Bicycle clothing

plate built in to achieve that sole stiffness. This helps distribute the pedaling force over a large area of the foot. Consequently, the pressure at any one point of the foot is within the comfortable range, and a more efficient transfer of energy from the legs to the bicycle drivetrain results.

Bicycling shoes either have metal or plastic cleats or a patent clamping device similar to a miniature ski binding, to hold the feet in place on the pedals. There is little doubt that either system allows more secure pedaling, especially on long trips where there is rarely a need to get off the bike. However, these things make it nearly impossible to walk, and tricky enough to get on and off.

If you're out to do more things than just riding your bike, you will probably want to be able to walk in reasonable comfort as well. That not only rules out all most clipless binding systems, but also makes old fashioned cleats highly inconvenient. Either you do without cleats or you should have a spare pair of shoes easily accessible for getting around when off the bike.

In addition to the real things, compromise solutions in the form of walking/cycling shoes exist these days. They have stiff, slightly profiled plastic soles and well ventilated uppers. The cloth uppers unfortunately cause your feet to get saturated almost instantaneously in the rain — more about that under *Rain Gear* below. Similarly, cycling in cold weather poses special problems, which will also be covered separately.

Whatever kind of shoes you wear, they must have the right length and width not to hurt. Pull the shoe laces relatively tight in the upper part of the closure, so that the toes do not slip forward, getting pushed against the front of the shoe. Inside the shoes, choose cotton or wool socks that absorb perspiration. To be comfortable, they should be relatively thick, especially in the sole, and they should not have a knotty seam

in the toe area. If you wear street clothes, get socks that are long and elastic enough to fit over your pants legs to keep them out of the chain.

Shorts and Tights

Specific bicycle shorts are tight but stretchable knitted garments with rather long tight-fitting legs and a high waist. They generally stretch so elastically that they stay up without the need for a belt, though suspenders (braces to my British audience) may be required, depending on your body build. Sewn in the crotch area is a soft and smooth piece of chamois leather, which protects the skin against chafing and absorbs perspiration. Correctly worn directly over the bare skin, they must be washed out daily. Consequently, you need at least two pairs to make sure you always have a clean pair.

Old fashioned woollen shorts and tights have the advantage that they regulate your body temperature better and get less smelly when they absorb perspiration. On the other hand, synthetics take up less moisture, dry a lot faster, and are much easier to wash.

One other way of minimizing the laundry problems is by wearing very light, stretchy seamless underpants underneath the cycling shorts. These items are available as regular women's underwear or may be obtained in men's versions from some bicycle outfits. They are much easier to wash out, quicker to dry and perfectly comfortable to wear.

In addition to ordinary bicycle shorts and tights —long legged cold weather versions of these same things —, there are special bicycle touring shorts and slacks that are quite practical if you're prepared to look less like a purist.

They can only be comfortable if they are smooth and soft. Stretchable materials are best and they should have no bulky seams. Slacks must be tight enough around the lower leg not to get caught in the chain. If they are not quite tight enough there, tuck the legs inside your socks or keep them together by means of elastic straps with a Velcro closure.

Shirts and Jerseys

The bicycling shirt or jersey is a tight fitting knitted garment with short sleeves, a very long bodice and pockets sewn on in the back. It works well to absorb perspiration, covers the parts of the torso that should be covered even when bending over, and doesn't flap in the wind. Similar things with long sleeves are designed for colder weather. Both long and short sleeved cycling shirts are available in wool and various synthetics. The former material is really most comfortable in colder weather or in e.g. hilly regions where temperatures may vary depending whether you're going uphill or down.

When it gets cooler, you may either wear a regular long sleeved cycling jersey or a thin, tightly fitting sweater over the top. Except in really cold weather, get a model that can be opened at the neck by means of a zipper. You may also wear a light windproof jacket over the top of your cycling shirt, providing it is made of a densely woven material that allows air and perspiration through.

Gloves

Even in warm weather, special cycling gloves are highly recommended, since they make the ride a lot more comfortable. This applies especially to riders who select a low riding style, which places a rather high percentage of their weight on the hands. These gloves have leather insides and open knit top panels and have fingers cut off to a length of about an inch. The palm area should be padded. If you do not like to wear gloves, at least use foam handlebar sleeves instead of (or underneath) regular handlebar tape, since this also provides the kind of cushioning effect needed to prevent nerve damage in the area of the palms. For colder weather, special winter cycling gloves are available, as will be described in a separate section below.

Head Protection

Back in the sixties and early seventies, head protection might at best have meant something to keep the rain off your head. Today, at least American and Australian cyclists have ample choice of real accident protection for their heads. In other countries the hard shell helmet, as it is generally called, is taking a long time to get established. I suggest you wear one, though I'll be the last person in the world to suggest making helmets mandatory: you're the person to decide what to do with your head. Meanwhile, refer to Chapters 5 and 6 for more details on the safety aspect of head protection.

Today's bike helmets all satisfy the elementary criteria. The most comfortable ones are the lightest. Fashion has played a role here too, with the unlined styrofoam models with separate fabric cover leading the way. These things are comfortable to wear, well ventilated, and attached so that they do not move out of place upon impact. Most of these important criteria are satisfied if the helmet meets the American standard ANSI Z-90.4. Many helmets can be combined with a shield or visor to keep the sun out of your eyes or the rain off your glasses.

There is one situation where a helmet

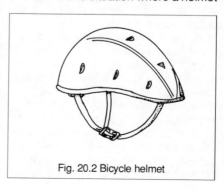

Fig. 20.2 Bicycle helmet

becomes too uncomfortable to wear for most people. That happens on a steep climb in hot weather. This situation is characterized by a combination of pro fuse perspiration, due to the heat generated as the result of performing work close to your maximum output, with the low speed that virtually precludes natural ventilation induced by air movement. I simply take off the helmet in a case like that. Just don't forget to put it back on as soon as the descent begins.

Rain Gear

Yes, it is entirely possible to ride a bike in the rain, even if it is 'only' in pursuit of fitness. In my native Holland you'd never get very far if you'd stop for every shower. Yet more people ride bikes there than anywhere else in the western world. Besides equipping the bike to keep the rain and spray off your body and the bike, you can make sure to have clothing that will see you through a heavy shower in reasonable comfort.

For the short pure fitness ride, there is an easy solution, acceptable as long as the temperature is above about 60°F (18°C): get wet. Once you get home, you can wipe yourself and put dry clothes on. However, for longer rides, and for lower temperatures, you will need special rain gear. Both this kind of clothing and the material described for cold weather cycling in the next section justify the perusal of a couple of bicycle mail order catalogs. Most of these companies have a summer and a winter catalog, the latter one often containing lots of useful items in this field, complete with worthwhile information on the properties of various materials and designs.

Fig. 20.3 illustrates some typical rain garments. The big problem is that perfectly waterproof materials don't only keep rain out, but also perspiration in. Even if you are not usually aware of it, the cyclist is continuously perspiring as a result of performing the work necessary to propel his machine. Normally, this perspiration evaporates immediately as it is absorbed by the air passing along the body. When an impermeable barrier in the form of rubber- or plastic-coated fabric prevents this natural process, the moisture condenses on the inside of the barrier and very soon it penetrates every fiber between your body and the rain gear, until you are as dismally soaked as you would have been without rain gear.

The only satisfactory solution to this dilemma is the use of a special material that is just porous enough to pass water vapor, without allowing the passage of liquid water. One material that satisfies this criterion is Goretex, a trade name for a cloth consisting of woven fabric with a barrier layer of stretched PTFE. There are a few other materials and coatings that do the same after a fashion, varying widely in price, weight and appearance.

Although most garments made with these materials are awfully expensive and often garishly styled, I consider the investment absolutely essential in most climates at any time, and at least for off-season cycling in more blessed regions. Available are jackets, capes, coats, pants and suits, designed either specifically for cycling or for general use. Try a number of different models out in a cycling or backpacking store, to make sure you get items that are not so generously cut as to hinder you while cycling.

Personally, I find the rain cape is still the best solution, provided it is combined with spats. The latter are a kind of leggings that are open in the back. They may be either home-made or purchased from the only known source of these things in the US, Custom Cycling Fitments. The cape should preferably be a model without a built-in hood, since the hood restricts your peripheral vision, which is especially important when checking behind before turning off. The best thing to keep your head dry is a helmet without vent holes — or a model with a rainproof liner.

Finally, with regard to rain gear, the feet are a real problem. Cycling shoes are little use when it comes to keeping your feet dry on a longer ride. This applies especially if a constant jet is being thrown up from the front wheel, as will happen when you have not installed fenders with a mud flap on the one for the front wheel. To ward off the rain from above, you may find good spats, with long beak-shaped extensions that reach over the tops of the shoes, quite effective. Another solution is to simply wear plastic bags around the socks, inside the shoes: not very elegant, but remarkably effective.

Cold Weather Wear

To be comfortable on the bike in cold weather, you will not need quite so much in the way of clothing as you would standing around watching a soccer game or waiting for your wife or husband. In the first place, the cycling activity generates enough heat to keep at least your trunk reasonably warm. In the second place, all that gear would hinder your movements. The heat is mainly generated in the trunk and the upper legs, so these parts will keep warm more easily, while the extremities of ears, hands and feet may need much thicker clothing.

Since the relatively high speed at which the cyclist proceeds causes high resultant air velocities, excessive wind chill may ensue in many cases. That is especially critical during descents, when the speed is high and your output low. Besides, even in summer it may get quite cold at high elevations. Consequently, bicycling in the mountains will cause additional problems, since you will be experiencing all the extremes. You'll be exposed to warm weather in the valleys and cold weather on the peaks, hard heat-producing cycling without significant wind cooling when climbing, and cold fast air-cooled descents.

To arm yourself for that, dress in layers that are easily put on and taken off. In addition, the wind must be kept out, for which a wind-proof outer layer is needed. That means a rather closely fitting, long jacket, made of very densely

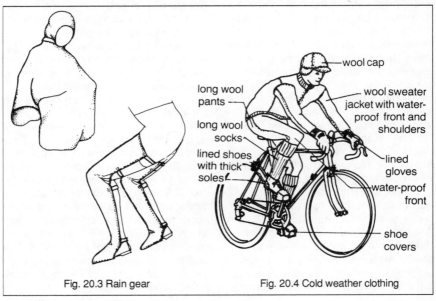

long wool pants

long wool socks

lined shoes with thick soles

wool cap

wool sweater jacket with water-proof front and shoulders

lined gloves

water-proof front

shoe covers

Fig. 20.3 Rain gear   Fig. 20.4 Cold weather clothing

woven cloth that is permeable to water vapor, preferably in two-layer construction. This same kind of outer shell also protects you best in winter, when winds seem to cut right through the warmest woollen wear.

Underneath this outer layer, wear several relatively thin layers of other warm materials. Quite close fitting knitted or other very stretchable materials are ideal. For long underwear, polypropylene is a good solution, since it is very light and not as hard on the skin as many other synthetics and wool. As for design, all these garments must be long, close fitting and easy to put on or take off. Zippers and other closures should be installed in such a way that there is a large enough overlap to keep the cold out, especially in the front.

Hands and feet cause greater problems, since the body's thermostat turns off the supply of heat-carrying blood to these extremities whenever the temperature of head and trunk is in danger of falling below the vital organs' required minimum operating temperature. Thick woollen socks inside special thick-soled and lined winter cycling shoes keep the feet comfortable. Add plastic bags, as described above for rain wear, if the combination of cold with rain or sleet occurs. Alternately, you may find pedal covers keep the feet comfortable under such conditions. Nylon backed woollen gloves or relatively light lined leather models, such as cross-country

skiing gloves, may suffice for the hands. Thick lined mittens may be needed when it gets even colder.

For the head, finally, a helmet without air scoops will be most comfortable, or a rainproof helmet cover for a model with. Makes you wonder why they put those silly holes in most helmets in the first place, because there are better methods of providing ventilation. In very cold climates, you may want to wear a thin cap underneath the helmet to cover the ears and other exposed portions of your head. And if you elect not to wear a helmet, you can get a knitted wool cap of the type shown in Fig. 20.4.

Though hard to find in the US, there are specific winter riding garments of the kind that is readily available in traditional cycling countries like France and England. If you should ever get there on your travels, don't forget to stock up on such useful things while you get the chance. These garments are integrated items that combine the warm materials in a design specifically intended for cycling, with wind breaking panels in the front of jacket and pants. Fig. 20.4 shows a cyclist wearing such gear. In addition, there are special add-ons to normal cycling garments that can be put on or taken off easily, although they look awful. These are particularly convenient at times and in areas where significant temperature differences maz be encountered in the course of a day's ride, such as in coastal and hilly regions.

Appendix

Table 1 Frame size determination

Leg length (measured per Fig. A)		Frame size (measured per fig. B, dimension X) Racing bike		Mountain bike	
cm	inches	cm	inches	cm	inches
73	29	43		35	14
74		44		36	
75		45	18	37	
76	30	46		38	15
77		47		39	
78		48	19	40	
79	31	49		41	16
80		50		42	
81	32	51	20	43	17
82		52		44	
83		53	21	45	
84	33	54		46	18
85		55		47	
86	34	56	22	48	19
87		57		49	
88		58	23	50	
89	35	59		51	20
90		60		52	
91	36	61	24	53	21
92		61		54	
93		62		55	
94	37	63	25	56	22
95		64		57	

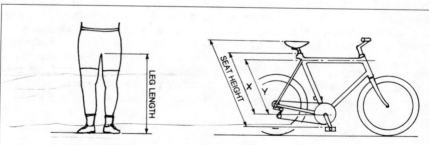

Fig. A. Inseam leg length determination   Fig. B. Frame size determination

Table 2. Gear Table in inches

number of teeth sprocket

number of teeth chainwheel

chainwheel \ sprocket	12	13	14	15	16	17	18	19	20	21	22	23	24	25	26	28	30
56	126	1163	108	1008	945	889	84	795	756	72	687	657	63	604	581	54	502
55	1237	1142	106	99	928	873	825	781	745	707	675	645	618	594	571	53	494
54	1215	1121	1041	972	911	857	81	767	729	694	662	636	607	583	56	52	486
53	1193	110	1022	954	894	841	795	753	715	681	65	622	596	572	55	511	475
52	117	108	1003	936	878	826	78	739	702	669	638	61	585	562	54	50	468
50	1123	1039	964	90	844	794	75	711	675	643	614	587	563	54	519	482	45
49	1102	1018	945	882	827	778	735	694	662	63	601	575	551	529	509	472	44
48	108	997	926	864	81	762	72	68	648	617	589	563	54	518	499	463	432
47	1057	976	906	846	793	746	705	666	634	604	576	552	529	508	488	453	421
46	1035	955	887	828	776	731	69	653	621	591	565	54	518	497	478	444	414
45	1012	934	867	809	76	715	675	64	608	579	552	528	507	486	467	437	405
44	99	914	849	792	743	699	66	625	594	566	54	516	495	475	457	424	396
42	945	872	81	756	709	667	63	597	567	54	515	493	473	454	436	405	375
40	90	831	771	72	675	635	60	568	54	514	491	47	45	432	415	386	36
38	855	789	733	684	641	603	57	54	513	489	466	446	428	41	395	366	342
36	811	747	695	648	609	572	54	511	487	464	442	424	405	389	374	348	324
34	765	706	655	611	572	54	51	482	459	437	416	399	382	367	353	328	306
32	72	664	617	576	54	508	48	455	432	411	392	375	36	346	332	308	286
30	675	623	578	54	506	476	45	426	405	386	368	352	337	324	312	289	27
28	63	581	54	504	472	444	42	397	378	36	343	328	315	302	29	27	251
26	585	54	501	468	437	412	39	368	351	334	319	305	292	28	27	25	232
24	541	498	462	432	405	381	36	341	324	308	294	281	27	259	249	231	216

Table 3. Gear conversion table: gear in inches to development in meters

Gear number (inches)

30	40	50	60	70	80	90	100	110	120	in

2,0	3,0	4,0	5,0	6,0	7,0	8,0		10,0	11,0	m

Development (meters)

Index

abrasions, 39
acceleration, 23 - 24
accessories, 103f
accidents, 34f
advantages of cycling, 7
aerobic, 69f
aerobic exercise, 8f
aerobic output, 76f
aerobic training, 76, 80, 83
age and cycling, 7
anaerobic, 70f
anaerobic threshold, 77
anaerobic training, 78, 81
annual training plan, 97f
ATP, 51, 57, 65
ATP-CP cycle, 51, 71

back ache, 41
bags, 126
balancing technique, 19f
basic fitness schedule, 100
basic fitness training, 8, 100
beta-endorphine, 71
bike accessories, 125f
bike clubs, 9
bike computer (also
    speedometer), 124
bike handling, 18
bike manufacturers, 105
bike parts, 114f
bike racing clothing, 132f
bike selection, 102f
bike types, 103f
Biopace chainrings, 119
blood glucose level, 72f
body fat, 62, 65
body temperature, 67
bonk, 71 - 72
bottom bracket, 118f
brain injury, 39
brake adjustment, 123
brake blocks, 122 - 123
brake levers, 122 - 123
brake test, 68, 123
brake types, 122f
brakes, 122f
braking technique, 17, 21
breathing exercises, 90
British v. American terms, 10
bronchial problems, 42

caffeine, 67
calcium (in food), 64
calisthenics, 82, 88
calories, 61, 65f
carbohydrate loading, 67

carbohydrates, 62
cell building (food), 61f
centuries, 10
century training schedule,
    100
chain, 119f
chain removal, 119
chain routing, 122
chain tool, 119
chainrings (also
    chainwheels), 119f
choice of path, 35
climbing, 25
clipless pedals, 133
clothing, 132
cogs (also sprockets), 121
cold weather, 135 - 136
cold weather clothing, 136
compensation effect, 74
constant speed riding, 23
control method, 82, 86
control method training, 86,
    93
cooling off, 83
cotterless crank, 119
crank tightening, 118
crankset, 118
cyclo-computer, 126
Cyclo-Simulator, 125

deceleration, 21
dehydration, 72
depletion, 74
derailleur, 121f
derailleur adjustment, 32
derailleurs, 28f, 103f
development (gearing), 31
development period, 98
digestion times, 65
diverting accidents, 37
drafting (also echelon), 24,
    27
drivetrain, 103f, 118f

efficiency, 43, 46, 58, 65
electrolytes, 72
endurance, 69
endurance training, 79
energy, 69f
energy from food, 61 - 62, 65
energy loss (walking v.
    cycling), 43
enzyme household, 71
enzymes, 61, 71
equipment, 124f
ergometer test, 51

ergometer training, 93
extender, 59

falls and collisions, 36f
fast twitch muscle fibers, 56
fat (as energy source), 65f
fats (food), 62f
fenders (also mud guards),
    126
FFA (free fatty acids), 63, 65
fibers (in food), 65
fit of bike, 11f
fitness bike (also sports
    bike), 104
fitness equipment, 124
flat (also puncture), 116f
flexor, 59
food, 61f
food requirements, 61f
food types, 61f
foot position, 14
force training, 81f
forced turn, 20
fractures, 39
frame, 102f, 107f
frame details, 107f
frame dimensions, 110f
frame geometry, 108
frame materials, 108
frame size, 110
frame tubing, 109
freewheel, 121
friction resistance, 45
front fork, 111

gear designation, 31f
gear selection, 32f
gearing, 28f
gearing practice, 30f
gearing system, 28f, 103,
    121
gearing theory, 29
getting on and off, 17
getting up to speed, 23
gloves, 134
glucose, 65f
glycogen, 65f
glycogen depletion, 72
gravitation effect, 44, 45
group riding, 9, 25, 27

handlebar adjustment, 15f
handlebar height, 15
handlebar position, 15
handlebar sleeves, 134
handlebar stem, 112

handlebars, 15, 12
handling technique, 16, 18
hard training schedule, 100
head injury, 39
head protection, 39, 134
headset, 111
health problems, 39f
health risks, 8f
heart rate (also *pulse*), 8, 76, 84
helmet, 134
helmet cover, 137
home trainer (also see *ergometer*), 125
honking, 25
hub, 103f
hybrid bike, 103

indexed gearing, 31f
indoor training, 88f
inner tube, 116
intermediate training plan, 99
interval training, 81, 84 - 85
isometric muscle use, 60

jersey, 134
jogging, 7
jumping the bike, 27

kJ (kilojoules), 65
knee problems, 41

lactic acid, 71, 77
lean angle (steering), 19f
leg muscle training, 80f
lighting, 35
liquids, 62
lock, 130
long range training plan, 97f
loss-off-control accidents, 38
LSD training, 83
luggage rack, 126
lunch, 68

mass, effect of, in acceleration, 47
massage, 94
materials, 108f
meal planning, 68f
mechanical friction, 45
minerals (food), 64
mountain bike, 104
mud guards (see *fenders*)
muscle efficiency, 58f
muscle fibers, 56f
muscle operation, 55 - 56, 58
muscle strength, 57, 59
muscle training, 56 - 57, 59,

79 - 80, 90, 125
muscle types, 55
muscles, 54f
myofilaments, 56

natural turn, 19
neuropeptides, 71
nighttime accidents, 35
nighttime protection, 35
non-round chainrings, 119
non-standard bikes, 104
numbness, 41
nutrition, 61f

obstacle avoidance, 26
overcompensation, 74
overheating, 72
overload, 74
overtraining, 42, 76

pain, 71
pain threshold, 71
participation period, 98
parts of bike, 102f
pedal covers, 136
pedal force, 30
pedaling rate, 29 - 30, 32, 79
pedals, 120
periodized training, 75f
personalized training, 82, 96f
physical examination, 8
posture when riding, 11f
potassium (in food), 64
power, 45ff
power (or *force*) intervals, 85
power requirement (cycling and running), 43
preparation period, 98
protein requirements, 63
proteins, 63
pulse (also see heart rate), 8, 76f
pulse rate monitor, 124
pump, 128
puncture kit, 116

quality of bike, 105
quick-release hub, 103f

racing bike, 104
rain gear, 135
recovery, 74
reflectors, 128
relative risks, 34
resting period, 98
resting pulse, 76
restraining muscles, 80, 90
riding comfort, 11

riding technique, 23
rim, 115
roller training, 92
rolling resistance, 45, 114
RQ (respiratory coefficient), 66
running v. cycling, 43

saddle, 13f, 113f
saddle adjustment, 15
saddle angle, 15
saddle height, 13
saddle position, 14
saddle sores, 40
safety, 34f
seat post, 102, 113
self massage, 94
set-up of bike, 11ff
shifters, 121
shirts, 134
shoes, 132
shorts, 133
sinus problems, 42
skeletal muscles, 54f
skidding accidents, 37
slant board, 125
slow twitch muscle fibers, 56f
snacks, 68
socks, 132
spare parts, 131
specificity, 56, 58, 74, 79
speed calculation, 29
speed in power calculation, 45
speed intervals, 85
speedometer (also *bike computer*), 124
spelling, 10
spokes, 115
spoking pattern, 115
sports bike, 104
sports drinks, 67
sprained limbs, 39
sprockets (also *cogs*), 121
starches, 62
steering geometry, 111f
steering system, 102f, 110f
steering technique, 18f
stem size selection, 16
stopping accidents, 36
stretching, 82, 88
sugars, 62
sun burn, 42
supper, 68

table salt, 64
technique training, 79, 82, 86
temperature, 67

tendinitis, 41
theft, 130
tire pressure gauge, 129
toeclips, 133
tool pouch, 131
tools, 131f
touring bike, 104
traffic hazards, 34f
traffic rules, 35
training effects, 73f
training log, 96
training methods, 83f, 88f
training periods, 97f
training plan, 96f
training pulse, 9, 84

training schedules, 99f
training specificity, 74f
training theory, 73f
triathlon bike (also *sports bike*), 104

valve types, 116, 129
vitamins, 63
$\dot{V}_{O2max}$, 51, 73, 75

warm-up, 83
warning device, 130
water, 62, 67, 72
water bottle, 129
weekly training plan, 99

weight training, 60, 81, 90
weight transfer in braking, 21
wet-weather braking, 22
wheel truing, 115
wheels, 103, 114
wind chill, 136
wind load simulator (also *turbo trainer*) training, 93
wind resistance (also *air resistance*), 11, 45
wind, riding against, 24
women v. men, 10, 71, 106
work (also see *energy*), 44f

Ordering books published by Bicycle Books, Inc.

All books published by Bicycle Books, Inc. may be obtained through the book or bike trade. If not available locally, use the coupon below to order directly from the publisher. Allow three weeks for delivery.

Fill out coupon and send to: **Bicycle Books, Inc.**
PO Box 2038
Mill Valley CA 94941 (USA)
FAX (415) 381 6912

Please include payment in full (check or money order made out to Bicycle Books, Inc. or credit card info). If not paid in advance, books will be sent UPS COD.

Canadian and other foreign customers please note: Prices quoted are in US Dollars. Postage and handling fee for foreign orders is $3.50 per book ($4.50 Air Mail). International Money Order in US currency (enquire at Post Office) must be enclosed.

Please send the following books:

The Mountain Bike Book	___ copies @	$9.95	= $ ___
The Bicycle Repair Book	___ copies @	$8.95	= $ ___
The Bicycle Racing Guide	___ copies @	$10.95	= $ ___
The Bicycle Touring Manual	___ copies @	$10.95	= $ ___
Roadside Bicycle Repairs	___ copies @	$4.95	= $ ___
Major Taylor (hardcover)	___ copies @	$19.95	= $ ___
Bicycling Fuel	___ copies @	$7.95	= $ ___
Mountain Bike Maintenance	___ copies @	$7.95	= $ ___
In High Gear	___ copies @	$10.95	= $ ___
The Bicycle Fitness Book	___ copies @	$7.95	= $ ___
The Bicycle Commuting Book	___ copies @	$7.95	= $ ___
The New Bike Book	___ copies @	$4.95	= $ ___
Bicycle Technology	___ copies @	$16.95	= $ ___
The Tour of the Forest Bike Race	___ copies @	$9.95	= $ ___

Sub total	$ ___
California residents add sales tax	$ ___
Shipping and handling: $2.50 first book, $1.00 each additional book (within US)	$ ___
Total amount	$ ___

Name _____

Address _____

City, _____

State, zip _____   Tel. (___)_____

MC / VISA No. _____ Signature _____